Handbook of Paediatric Accident and Emergency Medicine

A SYMPTOM-BASED GUIDE

Handbook of Paediatric Accident and Emergency Medicine

A SYMPTOM-BASED GUIDE

Edited by

DMW Capehorn

Associate Director in Medico-legal Practice (Medico-legal Consultancy, Gloucester) and Clinical Assistant in Accident and Emergency Medicine, Worcester. Formerly Fellow in Paediatric Accident and Emergency Medicine, Royal Hospital for Sick Children, Bristol and former Trust Specialist in Accident and Emergency Medicine, Weston Area Health Trust, UK

AH Swain

Consultant in Accident and Emergency Medicine and Director of Accident and Emergency Service, Bristol Royal Infirmary, and Weston-super-Mare General Hospital, UK

LL Goldsworthy

Consultant Paediatrician with specific responsibility for Accident and Emergency and Ambulatory Paediatrics, Royal Hospital for Sick Children, Bristol, UK

W.B. Saunders

London • Edinburgh • New York • Philadelphia • Sydney • Toronto

W. B. Saunders is an imprint of Harcourt Brace and Company Limited

Harcourt Brace and Company Ltd 24–28 Oval Road
London NW1 7DX, UK

The Curtis Center
Independence Square West
Philadelphia, PA 19106-3399, USA

Harcourt Brace & Company
55 Horner Avenue
Toronto, Ontario M8Z 4X6, Canada

Harcourt Brace & Company, Australia
30–52 Smidmore Street
Marrickville, NSW 2204, Australia

Harcourt Brace & Company, Japan
Ichibancho Central Building, 22–1
Ichibancho, Chiyoda-ku,
Tokyo 102, Japan

© 1998 Harcourt Brace and Company Limited

This book is printed on acid free paper

A catalogue record for this book is available from the
British Library

ISBN 0–7020–2168–7

Typeset by J&L Composition Ltd, Filey, North Yorkshire
Printed and bound in Great Britain by WBC, Bridgend, Mid Glamorgan

CONTENTS

PART I   Dealing With Children

PART II   Emergency Ambulatory Presentations

FOREWORD

Some 20% of children attend Accident and Emergency services each year. Put another way, children account for approaching one third of the patients seen in A&E departments. And yet, paradoxically, it is only recently that Accident and Emergency Paediatrics has emerged as a discrete specialized subject: the tempo is quick, the work intensity infinitely variable and the clinical spectrum unlimited in its breadth.

The first steps in the handling of an emergency case can define the whole trajectory of the child's care and clinical outcome, affecting the soma and the psyche, the child and the family. Some children are critically ill and require immediate intensive care; others may appear well yet no child presents to an A&E department at midnight without a serious underlying if unobvious cause.

Those who work in hospital 'casualty' departments will greatly welcome the *Handbook of Paediatric Accident and Emergency Medicine*. It is timely, succinct and presented in a bullet point, box and list style which is easily accessible. It has been written from the real world of A&E Paediatrics, is symptom orientated and pragmatically practical. There is much wisdom in this text. The A&E practitioner will do well to have it readily to hand.

JD Baum
Professor of Child Health
University Department of Child Health, University of Bristol, and Consultant
Royal Hospital for Sick Children, Bristol, UK
November, 1997

PREFACE

There are many excellent textbooks of paediatrics but rarely do they address the need of those on the 'front line' of hospital care – primarily junior hospital doctors in the specialties of A&E Medicine and Paediatrics. Such professionals are often worried about the management of children, who tend to present with a 'symptom' (or collection of symptoms). This was the case in our own experience and in our own departments. A need was identified for a relatively short handbook outlining the management of the ill or injured child in the A&E department, which we hope this book fulfils.

Whilst the book was primarily aimed at junior hospital doctors it will also appeal to A&E nurses and nurse practitioners, general practitioners, paramedics and other allied personnel involved in the care of the acutely unwell or injured child.

We are indebted to a great many more people than we can possibly name. However, special praise must be reserved for the patience and support of our families, and the staff of WB Saunders. In particular our gratitude goes to our dedicated and unpaid typist, proof reader and critic, Fiona Capehorn.

DMWC
AHS
LLG
April 1998

CONTRIBUTORS

The following individuals are thanked for their help in the preparation of one or more chapters of the book:

Professor P Fleming
Professor of Infant Health and Developmental Physiology
Consultant Paediatrician
Institute of Child Health
Royal Hospital for Sick Children
Bristol, UK

Mrs M Griffin
Research Health Visitor
FSID Unit for Research into Infant Health and Development
Institute of Child Health
Royal Hospital for Sick Children
Bristol, UK

Dr D Heller
Staff Grade Paediatrician
Accident & Emergency Department
Birmingham Children's Hospital
UK
(Formerly Consultant in Community Paediatrics, Weston-super-Mare General Hospital, UK)

Dr G Hughes
Clinical Director Emergency and Trauma Services
The Emergency Department
Wellington Hospital
Wellington
New Zealand

Dr S Mather
Consultant in Paediatric Anaesthesia
Royal Hospital for Sick Children
Bristol, UK

Dr P Stoddart
Consultant in Paediatric Anaesthesia
Royal Hospital for Sick Children
Bristol, UK

ACKNOWLEDGEMENTS

We also offer special thanks to the following, all of whom offered specific help and advice or contributed material to the book:

Mr D Baldwin
Consultant Ear, Nose & Throat Surgeon
Southmead Hospital
Bristol, UK

Mr M Gargan
Consultant Orthopaedic Surgeon
Royal Hospital for Sick Children
Bristol, UK

Sr R Hoskins
Sister in Charge and Nurse Manager
Accident & Emergency Department
Royal Hospital for Sick Children
Bristol, UK

Dr C Kennedy
Consultant Dermatologist
United Bristol Health Care Trust
Bristol Royal Infirmary/Bristol Children's Hospital
UK

Mr R Spicer
Consultant Paediatric Surgeon
Royal Hospital for Sick Children
Bristol, UK

Dr J Tizzard
Consultant Paediatric Nephrologist
Southmead Hospital
Bristol, UK

Dr P Weir
Consultant Paediatric Anaesthetist and Intensivist
Royal Hospital for Sick Children
Bristol, UK

Dr C Williams
Senior Registrar in Ophthalmology
Bristol Eye Hospital
UK

Grateful thanks are also offered to the following individuals for their general help in the preparation of this book: John Tustin, Kay Cuff, Duncan Goodland, Maria Khan and the many others who have offered helpful comments.

HOW TO USE THIS BOOK

This book is essentially a practical tool. It is divided into sections. Within each section specific presentations are considered symptom by symptom. Wherever possible a standard format is followed within each chapter, as follows:

BACKGROUND INFORMATION

DIAGNOSTIC APPROACH   History

Examination

Investigations

MANAGEMENT AND REFERRAL

OUTCOME AND PROGNOSIS

Text that appears in **bold** indicates the need to **record** such information in the medical records. *Specific diagnoses* are recorded in *italics*.

Lists of *causes* of a symptom (for information) or condition are recorded in boxes such as that below:

Important information, *of which careful note should be made*, is recorded in shaded boxes such as that below:

Cross referencing to other chapters in a book such as this are inevitable, but we have tried to keep this to a minimum.

It is recommended that you read the chapters in Part 1 of the book as the principles applied will be of relevance to all other chapters.

Although the book is 'symptom based' we hope sufficient information will be found in the short notes of each condition to make the book stimulating.

LIST OF ABBREVIATIONS

A&E	Accident and Emergency (Medicine)
ASO	Anti streptolysin O
AVPU	Alert, (respond to) Voice, (respond to) Pain, Unresponsive
BP	Blood pressure
CRP	C-reactive protein
CT	Computerized tomography
CVP	Central venous pressure
CXR	Chest X-ray
DKA	Diabetic ketoacidosis
DMSA	Dimercapto-succinic acid
ECG	Electrocardiogram
EEG	Electroencephalogram
ENT	Ear, nose and throat
FBC	Full blood count
GCS	Glasgow coma scale
GOR	Gastro-oesophageal reflux
GP	General practitioner
HSP	Henoch–Schönlein purpura
ITP	Idiopathic thrombocytopenic purpura
iv	Intravenous
LMA	Laryngeal mask airway
LP	Lumbar puncture
LRTI	Lower respiratory tract infection
MC&S	Microscopy, culture and sensitivity
MCUG	Micturating cysto-urethrogram
MDI	Metered dose inhaler
MRI	Magnetic resonance imaging
NAI	Non-accidental injury
NPA	Nasopharyngeal aspirate
NSAIDs	Non-steroidal anti-inflammatory drugs
NSAP	Non-specific abdominal pain
PCR	Polymerase chain reaction
SIDS	Sudden infant death syndrome
U&E	Urea and electrolytes
URTI	Upper respiratory tract infection
UTI	Urinary tract infection
VZV	Varicella zoster virus

NOTICE

Every effort has been made to check the drug dosages given in this book. However, as it is possible that dosage schedules have been revised, the reader is strongly advised to consult the current *British National Formulary* or the drug companies' literature before administering any of the drugs listed.

PART I

Dealing with Children

1 INTRODUCTION

BACKGROUND INFORMATION

- In some hospitals over 90% of paediatric hospital admissions enter through the accident and emergency (A&E) department.
- Be relaxed in your approach to the child. Engage both child and carers during the consultation.
- Conduct the consultation in a room designed for children with pictures and toys available, as children will need these once they have tired of medical discussions between adults.
- If a child is obviously unwell, call for help while getting the initial details.
- Above all, remember that working with children can be fun!

DIAGNOSTIC APPROACH

History

- A thorough history is vital as this determines the diagnosis in most cases; examination and investigations merely lend supportive evidence.
- Use a standard history format, as for adult patients, but pay special attention to the points in Box 1.1.
- In addition, record in the notes whether the history was obtained **from the carer or the child**.

Box 1.1 *Key factors in a child's history*

HISTORY OF PREGNANCY, DELIVERY, PUERPERIUM, FEEDING METHODS

DEVELOPMENTAL HISTORY – in all children under 2 years old and in older children with neurological symptoms

HISTORY OF IMMUNIZATIONS – particularly important for parental education and serious pathogens (e.g. *Haemophilus influenzae*)

FAMILY HISTORY – e.g. a family history of asthma, febrile fits or diabetes

CONTACT WITH INFECTIOUS DISEASES – (including travel abroad)

SOCIAL HISTORY (vital!) – note who the carers are (e.g. lone parent, grandparents, etc.) and the home background (e.g. cramped accommodation); presentation of a 'well' child may represent the need for social support and is relevant to the prevention of non-accidental injury (NAI)

DRUG HISTORY – children are often taking 'over the counter' medicines or other prescribed medicines

Examination

- Examine babies and infants on the lap of the carer if possible.
- Get on your knees for small children!
- Explain to toddlers what you intend to do and then do it; older children can be asked for specific permission.
- As a general rule examine the part that presents to you, if possible starting away from any sensitive or painful area to gain confidence; save unpleasant procedures (e.g. examination of fauces) until last.
- All children should have basic observations recorded – at the very least **pulse**, **respiratory rate**, **temperature** and, in some instances, **blood pressure**. An accurate **weight** is helpful in determining drug dosages.
- In some cases, especially where there is a chronic underlying prob-

lem, an accurate record of **height** and **head circumference** may be helpful (e.g. a baby with developing hydrocephalus may have an enlarging head).

- It is often helpful to use a period of observation in the department (e.g. to watch for the progress of a pyrexia) and this may be used to complete areas of examination deferred on the first occasion.

Investigations

In the A&E department investigations are needed only:

1. To help make the diagnosis or influence treatment.
2. When samples are needed for culture or to provide baseline values before treatment.

Do not, however, be afraid to investigate in A&E when appropriate – time obtaining samples and waiting for results can be invaluable for observing children.

Practical advice about procedures such as venesection can be found in Part V.

MANAGEMENT AND REFERRAL

Management will accord with the diagnosis made but an attempt should be made to categorize the severity of the illness into mild, moderate or severe (see Chapters 2 and 3). Certain general points, however, should be remembered.

- Be more cautious the younger the child; infants are particularly difficult to assess clinically. Infants under 3 months should be treated very cautiously indeed.
- On the whole parents usually know when their children are very ill; listen to them!
- Remember that treatment is more important than investigations.
- Do not be pressured by time or workload into an 'instant' decision – use a period of observation in the department if possible. Refer for advice if in any doubt.

- Paracetamol suspension is essential in the armoury against pain and fever (dose according to the instructions on the bottle) – sick children have been known to revive when fever is controlled by paracetamol. Ibuprofen suspension is a widely used alternative.
- Drugs should be prescribed according to the doses given in an appropriate book (e.g. *Alder Hey Book of Children's Doses* – see 'Further Reading').

In general, the need for referral for advice (and possibly admission) will be determined by two factors:

1. The severity of the illness.
2. The parents' reaction to the illness and their home circumstances.

It is important to take into account both these criteria. Be ready to refer children who present to the department with the same symptoms on more than one occasion; there is always a reason, even if it is not always entirely medical!

In such circumstances:

Seek advice from senior A&E or paediatric staff!

OUTCOME AND PROGNOSIS

The outcome will depend on the diagnosis. There is no doubt that prompt intervention by properly prepared staff will improve the prognosis.

FURTHER READING

Alder Hey Book of Children's Doses. Sixth Edition (1994) Copies obtainable from Pharmacy Office, Royal Liverpool Children's Hospital (Alder Hey), Eaton Road, Liverpool L12 2AP.

2 ASSESSMENT OF THE UNWELL INFANT

BACKGROUND INFORMATION

The unwell infant is a difficult problem in the A&E department. It is important to differeniate the basically well infant with a transient viral infection from the unwell infant with more serious illness, including meningitis, urinary tract infection (UTI) and lower respiratory tract infection.

DIAGNOSTIC APPROACH

In a severely unwell infant call for help and conduct a primary survey:
Airway, breathing, circulation
Treat deficiencies as identified
Focus on important features in the history as you progress
(see Part III Chapter 1)

History

Ask about points listed below. Record:

- **Age**, **sex**.
- **Presenting complaint**: duration, mode of onset, severity (see Box 2.1); local or generalized problems.

Why has the patient been brought into A&E?
What treatment has already been given?
What are the parents' expectations?

- **History of pregnancy**, **delivery** and **puerperium**.

- **Developmental** progress.
- **Family history** of relevance.
- **Social history**.
- **Immunizations** completed to date.
- **Allergies, atopy**.
- **Past medical history** – any neonatal illness, other hospital atten-
  dances, history of weight gain, etc.
- Brief **systemic enquiry** – including history of **feeding** pattern.

The degree of severity of illness can be established by ascertaining the
answers to the questions in Box 2.1, which indicate the infant's general
well-being.

Box 2.1 *Establishing the severity of illness in an infant*

Is the baby alert and noticing surroundings?

Is the baby interested in feeds?

Is the baby playful?

Is the baby smiling?

Are there normal wet nappies? (four a day is a rough minimum)

If the answer to any of these is NO then beware!

Examination

- Bear in mind the general points made in Chapter 1.
- Check the nursing observations: **pulse, temperature, respiratory
  rate, blood pressure**.
- **General observations** – does the infant look well, ill or moribund?
- Examine the baby opportunistically but ensure top to toe evaluation
  is completed. Try to assess the cardiovascular and respiratory sys-
  tems and the abdomen while the baby is settled.
- **Fontanelle** – is it bulging (raised intracranial pressure, e.g. menin-
  gitis) or depressed (dehydration)?
- **Dehydration** if present may cause sunken eyes, sunken fontanelle,

dry mucous membranes, decreased skin turgor and loss of weight (see Chapter 7).

- **Ear, nose and throat** – remember to examine ears and throat in any febrile baby.
- **Skin** – examine the skin for rashes, bruising, swelling and reduced turgor, as part of a general examination as well as for any specific skin complaint.
- Respiratory system – look at the **rate** and **pattern** of breathing. Is there increased **work of breathing** (raised respiratory rate, flaring of alae nasi, expiratory grunt, nodding of head, diaphragmatic work causing abdominal protrusion)? Check the **effectiveness of breathing – colour, chest expansion, auscultation**.

  Note: In a normal infant the respiratory rate is 30–40 breaths min^{-1}. The ratio of pulse rate to the respiratory rate is approximately 4:1 so compare them. If the ratio is lower consider respiratory tract infection.
- **Circulation**: check **skin perfusion** – poor skin perfusion is suggested by

  slow capillary refill time (> 2 s after blanching for 5 s)
  pallor
  mottling
  cyanosis

  Check **pulse rate** and **character** (falling blood pressure is a late sign). Feel all major pulses (brachial and femoral) and note any delay or reduction in femoral pulse.
- **Abdomen** – inspect and gently palpate the abdomen. Percuss over any masses or areas of distension. Auscultate for the presence of bowel sounds. Check hernial orifices and external genitalia. The presence of a palpable liver edge is normal in infancy (1–2 cm).
- **Limbs** – observe whether all four limbs are used fully. Examine more closely where indicated.
- **Nervous system** – full neurological examination is rarely required. Observation of behaviour appropriate to the child's age is useful, e.g.

  focusing and smiling: 6 weeks
  reaching for objects: 4 months
  sitting and throwing toys: 8 months
  pulling to stand: 11 months

A rough guide to rousability can be obtained using the 'AVPU' scale.

ALERT
Responds to VOICE
Responds to PAIN
UNRESPONSIVE

Summary of history and examination

As a general guide, *simple* observations by the parents, nurses and doctor can lead to a straightforward classification of infants who are mildly, moderately or severely unwell (Table 2.1).

Table 2.1 *Severity of illness in an infant*

Mild illness	Moderate illness	Severe illness
Smiling	Miserable	Irritable or unconscious
Feeding, drinking	Irregular feeding pattern, reduced oral intake	Unable to feed
Interacting, playing	Uninterested in surroundings	Unresponsive
No cardiorespiratory compromise	Early changes in basic observations	Severe cardiorespiratory compromise

Note: Temperature is only a very rough guide, but if greater than 38.5 °C is a cause for concern in any child, particularly an infant.

Investigations

The investigations will depend upon the severity of the illness assessed according to Table 2.1. Investigations are summarized in Box 2.2.

Box 2.2 *General need for investigation*

> MILDLY UNWELL: probably no need
>
> MODERATELY UNWELL: investigate if diagnosis unsure or as a guide to treatment required.
>
> SEVERELY UNWELL: call for help immediately, resuscitate and investigate

Urine examination (microscopy and culture) is advised in any infant with significant, unexplained pyrexia (i.e. 38.5°C or over). This can be performed in a 'bag' specimen but a 'clean catch' is preferable (less risk of contamination). Skilled staff will sometimes perform a suprapubic aspiration of urine, if required (see Part V, Chapter 28).

In a moderately unwell infant, especially where the cause of illness is not obvious, investigations in the A&E department include:

- Urine for **urinalysis** and **microscopy, culture and sensitivities** (MC&S).
- **Full blood count**.
- **Urea and electrolytes, bicarbonate** and **blood glucose** measurements.
- **Blood cultures**.
- Consider **chest X-ray**.

MANAGEMENT AND REFERRAL

For a general guide, see Box 2.3.

Box 2.3 *Management and referral guidelines*

MILD ILLNESS: observe in the department if possible (e.g. to
check feeding regimens and observe response to antipyretics).
Treat the cause as appropriate. Refer to the general practitioner's
care, but advise to return if any deterioration occurs

MODERATE ILLNESS: treat the cause of illness as
appropriate. If there is uncertainty about diagnosis and
treatment of these babies, refer to senior A&E or paediatric staff.
Advice regarding longer-term management or follow-up of
patients may also be needed

SEVERE ILLNESS: call immediately for assistance. An infant
who appears to have collapsed with sepsis should be treated
with oxygen, fluid resuscitation (10–20 ml kg^{-1}) and broad-
spectrum antibiotics after performing as much as possible of a
septic screen (see Chapters 5 and 21)

OUTCOME AND PROGNOSIS

The outcome will depend upon the diagnosis. However, it will be
improved by prompt and appropriate intervention.

3 ASSESSMENT OF THE UNWELL CHILD

BACKGROUND INFORMATION

Childhood encompasses the period from infancy to adolescence: from total dependence to competence. Presentation therefore varies, but the following guidelines will help to ascertain the severity of illness in children of all ages.

DIAGNOSTIC APPROACH

In a severely unwell child call for help and conduct a primary survey:
Airway, breathing, circulation
Treat deficiencies as identified
Focus on important features in the history as you progress
(See Chapter 1)

Proceed at a more relaxed pace in mildly or moderately unwell children.

History

- Objective – in a young child (under 3–4 years) the history will be an objective account from carers.
- Subjective – in an older child, expect a subjective account of symptoms with additional information from carers.
- Use the history to help you decide not only what is wrong but also the severity of the problem.

Ensure the history is obtained from relevant sources
Record the source

Ask about the points listed below. Record:

- **Age, sex**.
- **Presenting complaint**: **duration, mode of onset, severity** (see Box 3.1), **local or generalized problem. Why have parents brought the child to be seen? What are their expectations?**
- **History of pregnancy, delivery** and **puerperium**.
- **Developmental history**: any neurological symptoms past or present.
- **Family history** of relevance.
- **Social history**: rough or detailed account depending on the nature of the presenting complaint.
- **Immunizations completed to date**: important in parental education and child health, in addition to being relevant to the management of important pathogens.
- **Allergies, atopy**.
- **Past medical history** – including any treatments already implemented and their effects, sources of medical advice, etc.
- **Brief systemic enquiry** – include eating, sleeping patterns, past ear, nose and throat (ENT) problems.

The degree of severity of illness can be established in young children by ascertaining the answers to the specific questions in Box 3.1.

Box 3.1 *Establishing the severity of illness in a young child*

Is the child smiling?

Is the child alert and interested?

Will the child play?

Is the child eating or drinking?

Examination

General points

See Chapters 1 and 2 for general points about examining young children.

- Check the nursing observations:
  pulse
  temperature
  respiratory rate
  blood pressure
- **General observations** – does the child look well, ill or moribund?

Specific observations

Examine opportunistically or, if possible, from top to toe. Gain the child's confidence by starting with simple observations. Explain what you are doing and why. Progress gradually to those areas perceived as more threatening.

- **Fontanelle** – if still present, is it bulging or depressed?
- **Dehydration** – may cause sunken eyes, dry mouth, ketotic breath, lack of tears when crying, reduced skin turgor (see Chapter 7).
- **Ear, nose** and **throat** – remember to examine ears and throat in any febrile child.
- **Skin** – examine the skin for rashes, bruising, swelling and reduced turgor, either as part of a generalized problem or in detail in a specific skin complaint.
- **Respiratory system** – look at the **rate** and **pattern** of breathing. Is there increased **work** of breathing (raised respiratory rate, flaring of alae nasi, expiratory grunt, use of accessory muscles)? Check the **effectiveness** of breathing – **colour, chest expansion, auscultation**.
- **Circulation** – check:
  capillary refill time (< 2 s is normal)
  pulse rate and **character** of the pulse
  blood pressure (falling blood pressure is a *late* sign, heralding imminent circulatory collapse)

The child who is genuinely shocked should be distinguished from one with peripheral vasoconstriction as a thermoregulatory response to fever

- **Abdomen** – inspect and then gently palpate the abdomen. Percuss as necessary over any masses or areas of distension. Auscultate for the presence of bowel sounds. Remember to examine hernial orifices and external genitalia. Rectal and vaginal examinations should be performed where indicated, but by the appropriate person and once only, if possible.
- **Limbs** – observe whether all four limbs are used fully. Examine carefully for tenderness, swelling, warmth, loss of movement around a joint, etc.
- **Nervous system** – full neurological examination is rarely required. Observation of movement during play is a useful approach to examination of the motor system. The degree of alertness can be tested using the 'AVPU' scale.

ALERT
Responds to VOICE
Responds to PAIN
UNRESPONSIVE

A modified Glasgow coma scale (GCS) (see p. 365) is available for use in younger children. The GCS score should be measured if conscious level is in doubt, e.g. after a head injury or seizure.

Severity of illness

In general, the older the child the easier it is to assess severity of illness. *Simple* observations by the parents, nurses and doctor can lead to a straightforward classification of children as mildly, moderately or severely unwell. With appropriate interpretation for age the simple guidelines given in Chapter 2 are applicable to children, especially younger children (e.g. pre-school) who can be more difficult to assess. These guidelines are reproduced in Table 3.1. below.

Table 3.1 *Severity of illness in a child*

Mild illness	Moderate illness	Severe illness
Smiling	Miserable	Irritable or unconscious
Eating, drinking	Irregular feeding pattern, reduced oral intake	Unable to eat or drink
Interacting, playing	Uninterested in surroundings	Unresponsive
No cardiorespiratory compromise	Early changes in basic observations	Severe cardiorespiratory compromise

Note: Temperature is only a very rough guide, but if greater than 38.5 °C is a cause for concern in any child.

Investigations

Investigations are required only where necessary to guide treatment or to assist in making a diagnosis in an unwell child.

> When time allows, apply local anaesthetic cream before venesection

If the child is *mildly unwell*, no investigations may be necessary. A **urine sample** for urinalysis and microscopy, culture and sensitivity (MC&S) should be considered in all, particularly if under an age where symptoms of dysuria might be reported (under 4 years). A **throat swab** for bacteriology and virology may be relevant.

If the child is *moderately or severely unwell* consider venesection (see Part V) for **blood glucose** estimation, **urea and electrolytes**, **blood cultures**, **full blood count** (FBC) and **C-reactive protein**, provided the tests are being done for the reasons indicated above. **Chest X-ray** may be indicated. **Urinalysis** and **urine** for MC&S is important and a **throat swab** may be indicated.

MANAGEMENT AND REFERRAL

Management will depend on the results of the evaluation performed.

Where possible, use time to help with your decisions. For example, if unsure whether to refer a child, observe while awaiting results of investigations and then reassess. Children with fever can revive when the temperature is controlled by appropriate doses of antipyretics.

Mild illness

Management may involve a period of observation of temperature (e.g. after administration of paracetamol) or feeding (if concerned about fluid intake). Referral back to the general practitioner (GP) to follow up the results of any investigations or the response to treatment is appropriate. Ask parents to obtain advice (from GP or A&E department) if there is any deterioration or change in symptoms.

Moderate illness

If a child is moderately unwell and the diagnosis or immediate prognosis is uncertain, an opinion from experienced A&E or paediatric staff should be sought. Referral for advice regarding management of a continuing illness may also be required, e.g. for further investigations following a UTI (see Chapter 8).

Severe illness

Treat immediately and call for assistance and advice.

OUTCOME AND PROGNOSIS

The outcome depends upon the underlying condition.

> With prompt treatment most seriously ill children have an
> excellent chance of recovery

Emergency Ambulatory Presentations

4 THE CRYING BABY

BACKGROUND INFORMATION

- Crying is the most common way in which an infant or young child communicates distress or need. In general, the younger the child, the more difficult it is to interpret the crying.
- Crying in the newborn may indicate hunger, thirst or discomfort. After 2–3 months infants may learn that thumbsucking soothes and smiling gets attention. By 6 months crying is used to attract attention. After this age, separation, frustration and boredom become significant factors in its genesis.
- Persistently crying babies are at increased risk of physical abuse (see Chapter 26). Crying varies from baby to baby but those who cry more may be oversensitive to situations of any sort. Parental anxiety increases and the crying can subsequently worsen. The 'vicious circle' then needs to be broken.
- There are two main problems in dealing with the crying baby:
  1. Diagnosis and treatment of physical illness or injury (typically these conditions present with *acute crying*).
  2. Help for the parents in managing a *persistently* crying baby (i.e. prolonged or *chronic crying*).
- A thorough clinical evaluation is required not only to exclude physical problems but also to relieve parents' fears of underlying serious illness. In all cases there remains the problem of defining what is excessive or frequent crying, and this may be as much dependent upon parental experience as factors within the child.

DIAGNOSTIC APPROACH

The general principles outlined in Chapter 2 should be observed. In addition, the following notes will be helpful in determining the cause of the crying.

History

A *full* history is *essential* if all relevant information is to be obtained. Although difficult in the circumstances, an attempt should be made to take the history in a methodical fashion.

Duration of crying

If the crying had its onset within the previous 24 hours, recent illness or injury are the likely causes. If the duration has been days or weeks, these are less likely.

Pattern of crying

- Intermittent episodes of inconsolable crying, associated with sweating and pallor, suggest conditions such as intussusception. Typically the pattern repeats every 10 minutes or so.
- Crying on swallowing or feeding may indicate an upper respiratory tract infection such as tonsillitis or otitis media.
- Crying on lying down may indicate oesophagitis.
- Crying when a bottle is placed into the child's mouth may suggest oral ulceration or thrush.
- Crying on movement may suggest musculoskeletal problems (e.g. joint or bone problems such as fractures or infection).
- Crying associated with bowel opening may suggest constipation or anal fissure; crying on passing urine may suggest a urinary tract infection.
- Crying out during handling suggests 'irritability' and may be an indication of meningism in a baby. In these cases, the cry may be high-pitched or whimpering.

Behaviour when not crying

Ask the parent how the baby behaves when not crying. An alert baby (his or her 'usual self') is unlikely to be unwell, but a baby who between bouts of crying is distressed or drowsy may be severely unwell.

Associated symptoms

Ask if any specific symptoms are present, for example vomiting, diarrhoea, cough or feeding difficulties, which may point to a particular diagnosis (see the relevant chapter in this book).

Previous history

- A recent history of immunization may be important. Screaming spells after pertussis immunization are well recognized and, if prolonged over 24 h, may be a contraindication to further immunization (discuss with a paediatrician).
- A recent history of infection in siblings may be relevant.
- A recent history of trauma, even if considered insignificant by the parents, should be sought.
- Previous treatment (tried by doctors and parents) should be ascertained and recorded.

Family history

Ask if this is the parents' first baby, or how the baby's crying compares with the parents' experiences of older children.

Examination

There is no substitute for a full examination as detailed in Chapter 2. Even in cases where no organic cause is suspected from pointers in the history, a full examination is reassuring for the doctors and parents alike.

- Observation of the baby both when crying and when responding to soothing is helpful.
- Each system should be examined in turn to look for signs suggestive of a specific diagnosis.
- Growth should be assessed for any child with chronic persistent crying, by referring to standard growth charts.
- A differential diagnosis may include some of the conditions outlined in Box 4.1.

Box 4.1 *Causes of acute crying*

INFECTION

ENT: e.g. otitis media, tonsillitis

CENTRAL NERVOUS SYSTEM: e.g. meningitis, encephalitis

GENITOURINARY SYSTEM: UTI

RESPIRATORY SYSTEM: e.g. pneumonia

MUSCULOSKELETAL: e.g. septic joint, bone infection

SKIN: e.g. pruritus due to scabies, nappy rash

GASTROINTESTINAL SYSTEM: e.g. gastroenteritis, stomatitis

NON-INFECTIVE CONDITIONS

ENT: e.g. pharyngeal abrasion, nasal obstruction

CARDIOVASCULAR SYSTEM: rarely heart failure, arrhythmias (e.g. supraventricular tachycardia)

GASTROINTESTINAL SYSTEM: e.g. oesophageal reflux, inguinal hernia, anal fissure, constipation, intussusception

GENITOURINARY SYSTEM: e.g. obstruction, retention of urine

MUSCULOSKELETAL: haematoma, fracture, joint inflammation (transient synovitis, arthritis)

SKIN: e.g. pruritus due to eczema or urticaria

CENTRAL NERVOUS SYSTEM: e.g. raised intracranial pressure (tumour, subdural haematoma)

OTHER: e.g. clothing threads around digits

Investigations

When the cause of acute crying is not evident on clinical assessment further investigation is warranted, which will depend on the presentation. In general terms:

- If *infection* is suspected a **full septic screen** may be indicated if the child is severely unwell (see Chapter 5). A mildly or moderately unwell and pyrexial infant presenting with acute crying should, at the very least, have a **urine specimen** examined.
- If *trauma* or a musculoskeletal disorder is suspected, **X-rays** may be indicated (see Chapters 15, 16 and 29).
- If *intra-abdominal* problems are suspected, **X-rays** or **ultrasound examination** may be useful, especially in the diagnosis of intussusception. **Barium** or **Air enema**, in a unit with suitable surgical support, can be used in both the diagnosis and treatment of the latter condition.

MANAGEMENT AND REFERRAL

Management will depend upon the diagnosis, but it is important to remember that an acutely unwell child should be properly resuscitated (see Part III) and provided with adequate analgesia, whether or not a definitive diagnosis has been made.

- At the end of a thorough history and examination, if there is any doubt about illness or injury being the cause of the baby's acute crying, obtain advice from senior A&E colleagues or a paediatrician.
- Many babies will have a completely normal examination and will appear well, with no symptoms of disease. In these instances only general advice can be given. Parents often find that rhythmic movement (e.g. a car journey) soothes a baby. Changes in feed are often tried, without good reasons, but there is sometimes coincidental improvement. Relatives and friends may be encouraged to take over the baby's care. The GP and health visitor should be informed and asked to provide community support. It is important to remember that the majority of crying babies settle spontaneously.
- Sometimes parents and babies become so distressed and exhausted that they cannot be sent home. Under such circumstances admission may occasionally be offered to relieve the acute situation, particularly if community support is not in place. In this way a potentially dangerous situation may be avoided.

- One diagnosis worth a specific mention is 'infantile colic'. This is a behavioural syndrome characterized by paroxysmal crying, particularly in the evenings, associated with drawing-up of the knees and without identifiable cause. It is a diagnosis made by exclusion of more serious disorders. The infants, typically aged a few weeks to a few months, are otherwise healthy. Relief occasionally occurs when the baby passes a stool or wind, and episodes become less frequent and less severe after 3 months of age. The children usually thrive and no medication has convincingly been shown to be beneficial. Many theories exist as to its causation; some relate to food allergy, some to abnormal gut motility, but none has been proved. The importance of the condition is that, once serious causes are excluded, reassurance can be given to the parent that the episodes of 'colic' will eventually settle.

OUTCOME AND PROGNOSIS

Outcome is dependent on the diagnosis. However, the majority of crying babies settle (eventually!) and help and reassurance should be offered to parents to bolster and not undermine their confidence.

5 CHILDREN WITH FEVER OR FEBRILE FIT

An acute febrile response is the most common presentation of illness in childhood. For some the first sign of illness may be a febrile fit. Guidelines to the systematic assessment of the unwell infant and child are given in Part I.

This chapter deals with the management of a child presenting with a febrile fit, but the principles are useful in assessing any child with unexplained fever. Management is directed towards identifying the cause and excluding serious infection (for example, meningitis, septicaemia). Often the fit has ceased by the time of presentation at the A&E department. Occasionally the fit may be prolonged, in which case initial management is directed towards resuscitation and stopping the fit (Chapter 19).

BACKGROUND INFORMATION

- *Definition – a febrile fit* is a tonic or tonic-clonic fit occurring in a child aged 6 months to 6 years, precipitated by fever, arising from infection outside the central nervous system, in a child who is otherwise developmentally normal.
- *Epidemiology* – febrile fits affect 2–5% of children under 5 years old, the male to female ratio being 2:1. There is a positive family history in up to a third of cases (e.g. sibling or parent). The mean age is 17–23 months. The majority of fits are described as 'simple' (80%), the remainder being 'complex'.

  A *simple* febrile fit is one that lasts for less than 15 min. It is not repeated in the same episode. There are *no focal features*, and recovery is complete within 1 h.

  A *complex* fit (20%) is either prolonged (over 15 min), focal or with incomplete recovery, for example Todd's paresis (in which there are persisting unilateral neurological signs beyond the immediate post-ictal phase). Prolonged febrile fits account for a quarter of all cases of status epilepticus in childhood.

Status Epilepticus is a single convulsion lasting longer than 30 min or a series of convulsions during which the patient does not regain full consciousness.

- *Temperature*: a rapid *rise* in temperature is said to be important but *at the time of the fit* 75% have a temperature over 39°C.
- *Aetiology*: the most common causes are viral illnesses (80–90%). Identifiable causes include upper respiratory tract infection (URTI), otitis media, lower respiratory tract infection (LRTI), urinary tract infection (UTI) and gastroenteritis. Fever following immunization *can* lead to a febrile convulsion (for example 7–10 days following measles vaccination).

DIAGNOSTIC APPROACH

Resuscitation

The priority is to stop the fit (Chapter 22) and stabilize the patient following the standard protocols (Chapter 19).

History

It is important to establish the following:

- **State of health prior to the fit**. Typically the child is only a little off-colour or completely well prior to the fit.
- **Features of the fit**. Obtain an accurate description of the fit, if at all possible. Any of the following features may be described by parents, but it is essential to establish whether *consciousness is lost*:
    the eyes may roll up
    the limbs may stiffen
    there may be cyanosis
    there may be generalized movement of upper and lower limbs
- **Previous medical history**. Any previous history of fits, febrile or afebrile, should be noted, as should contact with infectious disease or travel abroad.

- **Family history**. A family history of febrile fits or epilepsy should be documented. A positive family history of febrile fits is found in up to 30% of cases.
- **Medication**. The child may already be taking antibiotics or other medication for the illness.

Examination

The unconscious child should be assessed as outlined in Chapter 22. Briefly, this consists of a 'primary survey' ('ABC' and 'AVPU' assessments) and a 'Secondary survey'. Otherwise general examination should follow the guidelines in Chapters 2 and 3, looking for obvious signs of infection.

Investigations

All children should have continuous pulse oximetry during the fit and recovery phase. Investigation depends on three factors:

clinical findings
age of patient
type of fit

Age under 6 months

- Any child presenting to the A&E department with high fever under the age of 6 months should be treated cautiously; the younger the child, the greater the need for caution.
- By definition a fit occurring with fever in this age group is *not a febrile fit* – it must be considered a sign of central nervous system infection until proved otherwise.

The child should be treated as for *meningitis* (see Chapter 22). **Antibiotic** therapy must be commenced and urgent discussion with senior A&E staff or paediatricians is needed. Ideally, as much of a **septic screen** as possible should be carried out before treatment is commenced, but ANTIBIOTIC TREATMENT SHOULD NOT BE DELAYED while these samples are collected.

Age 6 months to 18 months

Children aged 6–18 months should be treated with caution as signs of serious infection are few. Follow the guidelines in Chapters 2 and 3.

- If the child is *severely unwell* a full **septic screen** should be carried out, after appropriate resuscitation measures (Chapter 19). ANTI-BIOTIC THERAPY SHOULD NOT BE DELAYED IF OBTAINING THESE SAMPLES PROVES DIFFICULT.
- If the child is *mildly or moderately unwell* the child should be observed closely and the following investigations arranged:

   urine microscopy (always)
   full blood count (possibly)

   Further investigation should be guided by continuing clinical review. A partial or full septic screen should be considered if the child fails to show clinical improvement after appropriate cooling measures (Chapter 21), particularly if any of the following features are present:

   the child looks 'toxic' or 'irritable'
   the child shows any sign of meningitis
   the child shows signs of drowsiness or delayed recovery from the fit
   the fit was complex

Age over 18 months

Older children are easier to assess clinically.

- If the child is *severely unwell*, investigations are carried out as for the severely unwell child under 18 months (i.e. a full septic screen is required).
- If the child is *mildly or moderately unwell*, clinical assessment is of greatest importance:
   1. Where there is an obvious source of infection after thorough clinical assessment, no further investigations are required.
   2. Where the source of infection is not obvious or the fit was complex, **urine microscopy** should be arranged and consideration

given to other aspects of the 'septic screen' (Box 5.1) as guided by clinical findings.

> A lumbar puncture should not be carried out on a patient with a reduced level of consciousness
> A CT scan should be considered prior to the lumbar puncture

The investigations are helpful in determining the cause of the fever, which is the main aim of investigation. They are equally applicable to both simple and complex fits. However, *complex* fits have an increased association with other conditions, such as epilepsy so consider additional investigations in the case of complex fits:

urea and electrolytes (on presentation)

calcium and magnesium (on presentation)

CT scan (urgency dependent upon clinical state)

electroencephalography (non-urgent, usually best delayed)

Box 5.1 *Septic screen*

A septic screen consists of a **full blood count, throat swab, blood cultures, urine microscopy and culture, chest X-ray** and **lumbar puncture** (LP). In addition, some serum should be saved for **viral titres**

Although not strictly part of the 'screen', blood is taken for measurement of **C-reactive protein** (CRP), **urea and electrolytes**, and **blood glucose** (essential)

Within the A&E department it would be appropriate to carry out *all* these with the exception of the LP, which should be carried out by experienced personnel (a 'partial' septic screen)

Urinalysis: do NOT rely on dipstick analysis of urine samples in children, particularly infants. All samples should be sent to the laboratory for urgent microscopy (see Chapter 8). Research suggests that the combined use of traditional urine reagent strips (for proteinuria) with sticks that test for nitrites and leucocyte esterase may be useful in identifying samples where UTI can be excluded without the need for microscopy.

MANAGEMENT AND REFERRAL

Following a febrile fit, it may be reasonable to send the child home if the following criteria are met:

1. **The fit was simple**.
2. **The child has fully recovered**.
3. **There is an obvious source of infection**.
4. **The child is not severely unwell**.
5. **The parents are not unduly anxious**.
6. **The child has a previous and/or family history of febrile fits**.

However, as a general rule, cases involving first febrile fits should be discussed with senior A&E colleagues or paediatricians as too should any case where there is doubt about the diagnosis.

All cases not fitting the above criteria should be discussed with paediatricians.

If the child is discharged from the A&E department, the following details should be considered:

- **Appropriate treatment for the infection, if any**.
- **Advice about keeping the child cool**:
    removing clothes
    paracetamol syrup 15 mg kg^{-1} every 4–6 h orally or per rectum
    and/or ibuprofen syrup 5 mg kg^{-1} every 6–8 h
- **An advice sheet should be given about febrile fits.**
- **Follow-up should be arranged within 24–48 h (normally GP or occasionally A&E).**

OUTCOME AND PROGNOSIS

The parents should be counselled fully (nearly all parents think their child is dying during a first febrile fit). They should be told:

- The recurrence risk is less than 30%; 1 in 6 have three fits or more.
- Most recurrences occur within 1 year of the first.

- There is often strong family history, so other siblings should be kept cool during illnesses.
- Simple febrile fits have no relationship to the development of epilepsy. Children having *complex* fits often have outpatient electroencephalogram (EEG) and neuro-imaging scans arranged after discharge and should always have a follow-up appointment arranged with a paediatrician, as there is some relationship to epilepsy – however, the majority of the investigations will be normal.
- The immunization schedule should *not* be changed because of a simple febrile fit.

6 CHILDREN WITH RESPIRATORY SYMPTOMS

Respiratory symptoms are common in childhood. A wide variety of disorders present in a similar manner, with a small number of symptoms and signs. The most common acute presentations are:

a. Cough (acute and persistent).
b. Cough with wheeze.
c. Stridor.

Each of these presentations is considered in turn; the section on cough and wheeze is further subdivided into presentation in those under 1 year old and those over 1 year old.

a. COUGH

BACKGROUND INFORMATION

- Cough is a very common symptom seen throughout childhood.
- Cough can be an acute development in a previously well child or can develop as an exacerbation of a chronic cough. Causes are listed in Box 6.1.

The commonest cause of a cough is acute bronchitis, which generally has a viral aetiology and is a frequent condition in young children.

Box 6.1 *Causes of cough*

ACUTE

INFECTION: bronchitis, croup, pneumonia, pertussis/pertussis
  syndrome*, tuberculosis

OTHER: asthma, aspiration/inhalation

CHRONIC

Asthma, recurrent aspiration, cystic fibrosis, left heart failure,
  psychogenic

*Whooping cough is caused by *Bordetella pertussis*. Pertussis syndrome is
  a description given to an illness clinically identical to whooping cough
  but with a different aetiology (e.g. adenovirus)

DIAGNOSTIC APPROACH

History

Use the history to determine aetiology. A full history should be recorded
(Chapter 1); note in particular:

- **Duration** – the duration of the cough gives some idea of the diagnosis (see Box 6.1).
- **Fever** is often persistently high (> 38.5°C) in bacterial pneumonia
  and mild (< 38.5°C) in acute viral pneumonia, or bronchitis.
- **Cough** is absent or dry in the initial stages of pneumonia, but
  fruity with a 'rattly' chest in bronchitis. Paroxysmal cough leading
  to occasional vomiting (particularly at night) is characteristic of
  pertussis and pertussis syndrome. Apnoea may occur in infants.
  Recurrent discrete episodes of cough lasting a few days suggest
  asthma. Barking cough suggests croup.
- **Prodromal illness** – a URTI often develops 2–3 days before bronchitis or 2–3 weeks before pertussis, the paroxysmal cough developing in week 2. **Lethargy** and **fever** are more marked in bacterial
  pneumonia.
- **Pain** – pleuritic pain and abdominal pain may be features of
  pneumonia.

Examination

- **Temperature** – fever is high (> 38.5°C) in pneumonia, but absent or mild otherwise.
- **Pulse** – tachycardia occurs in pneumonia and after coughing paroxysms in pertussis syndrome.
- **Respiration** – the respiratory rate is increased when gas exchange is impaired, e.g. in pulmonary consolidation.
- **Work of breathing** – increased respiratory rate, flaring of nostrils and an expiratory grunt suggest increased respiratory effort (e.g. pneumonia). Intercostal recession and subcostal recession may also be features of pneumonia. In bronchitis and whooping cough, the work of breathing is not usually increased.
- **Effects of breathing** – loss of colour during a paroxysm in whooping cough is not uncommon, but the desaturation in acute pneumonia is persistent but not always clinically evident.
- **Chest movement** – may be reduced in area of decreased aeration in pneumonia.
- **Auscultation** – *crackles or other added sounds may or may not be present in pneumonia*. Moist crackles audible throughout chest occur in bronchitis, transmitted usually from mucus in the large airways. Dullness and decreased air entry in a child who has signs and symptoms of pneumonia often arise from a secondary pleural effusion. The lungs are usually clear in pertussis.

Increased respiratory rate and fever in an unwell child may be the only signs of pneumonia

- **Cardiovascular examination**: a persistent dry cough is common in left ventricular failure and may be the presenting symptom in children with cardiomyopathy. Clinical examination of the cardiovascular system will usually make the diagnosis clear.

Investigations

Investigations are not usually necessary but the following may be considered:

- **Pulse oximetry**.
- **Chest X-ray** when pneumonia is suspected or when cough persists or recurs for weeks.
- **FBC** is rarely helpful. Lymphocytosis (often $> 20 \times 10^9 \, l^{-1}$) supports a diagnosis of pertussis. Neutrophilia may occur in pneumonia.
- **Pernasal swab** may allow bacteriological confirmation of whooping cough.
- **Sputum culture** is occasionally helpful, particularly in older children, in the diagnosis of bacterial conditions.

MANAGEMENT AND REFERRAL

- If the child is hypoxic – give oxygen (see Chapter 20).
- Reassure parents of a basically well child with a cough. Antibiotics are not indicated but are often given for bronchitis.
- Once whooping cough has developed, eradicating the causative organism is not relevant but erythromycin may decrease the severity of the infection.
- Give a non-steroidal anti-inflammatory drug (NSAID), e.g. ibuprofen or diclofenac, for pleuritic pain. These drugs should be prescribed with care in a wheezy child.
- Give antibiotics in the mildly (or moderately) unwell child with pneumonia (usually penicillin, amoxycillin, co-amoxiclav or erythromycin).

Refer if the child is severely unwell, requires oxygen, has a poor oral intake, or is young (infant). An infant with suspected pertussis should also be referred for advice, because of feeding difficulties and increased risk of apnoea.

Children with persistent cough and failure to thrive should be referred. Further inpatient management includes:

> oxygen
> intravenous (iv) antibiotics in the severely unwell or vomiting child
> iv fluid (if vomiting)
> Ventilation is rarely required – usually for widespread viral pneumonia, occasionally for staphylococcal pneumonia.

OUTCOME AND PROGNOSIS

- Most children with bacterial pneumonia make a full recovery but deaths still occur, particularly when there is an underlying abnormality (for example, congenital heart disease).
- The cough of whooping cough may persist for weeks. Subconjunctival (and even periorbital) haemorrhage may result from paroxysms. Bronchiectasis may follow.

The common causes of acute cough are discussed below.

PNEUMONIA

Background information

- Pneumonia is *viral* in 90% cases; bacterial infection is more common in the older child.
- The type of organism and presentation will depend on age (Table 6.1).

Diagnostic approach

The typical presentation is as follows.

History

- **Prodromal illness** (sore throat, coryza) with **lethargy**.
- **Fever**, **cough**, **tachypnoea**, **cough** often dry then becoming looser.
- **Purulent sputum** in children over 5 years (unusual below this age).

Examination

- **Tachypnoea**, **respiratory distress** and **grunting** respiration are typical.
- **Dullness to percussion**, **decreased breath sounds**, **bronchial breathing** (but these signs may be absent, especially in younger children).

Table 6.1 *Causes of pneumonia in different age groups*

Age of child	Viruses	Bacteria
Neonatal	Respiratory syncytial virus	*Escherichia coli*, *Pseudomonas*, group B haemolytic streptococci, *Chlamydia* (rare but increasing)
Infancy (< 1 year)	Respiratory syncytial virus, parainfluenzavirus, adenovirus, rhinovorus, influenza virus, measles virus, varicella zoster virus (chicken pox)	*Staphylococcus aureus*, *Streptococcus pneumoniae*
Toddler (1–3 years)	As infancy	*Streptococcus pneumoniae* (90%); occasionally *Mycoplasma pneumoniae* (*Haemophilus influenzae* type b becoming rarer)
School age (4+ years)	Adenovirus, parainfluenza virus, influenza virus, cytomegalovirus, measles virus	*Streptococcus pneumoniae*; *Mycoplasma pneumoniae*

- **Abdominal pain** (lower lobe pneumonia), **neck stiffness and pleuritic chest pain** can also occur (pleural inflammation), sometimes referred to the shoulder tip.

Investigations

- **Radiography** is nearly always indicated when pneumonia is suspected because the classical signs of consolidation may be absent. As a general guide – any moderately unwell child with a cough and fever should have a chest X-ray (CXR).
- A CXR will confirm the extent and site of infection and the presence of complications (e.g. pleural effusion, lung abscess).
  Note: It is unusual to require a lateral film but left lower lobe collapse/consolidation can be overlooked on a posterior anterior view.

- Monitoring of **oxygen saturation (Sao$_2$)** should be mandatory where there is evidence of respiratory distress; **arterial blood gas analysis** is needed if the child is very ill.
- An **FBC** should usually be performed. Neutrophil leucocytosis is common in bacterial pneumonia.
- **Urea and electrolytes (U&E)** should be assessed in severe pneumonia; dehydration may be apparent and inappropriate ADH release may cause hyponatraemia.
- **Blood for culture and virology studies** (and possibly **sputum culture** in older children) aid in identification of infective organisms.

Management and referral

- The need for admission will depend on a number of factors including:
    age of patient (more caution required in younger patients)
    social circumstances, parental anxiety
    degree of distress
    need for iv treatment (see below)
- As a general guide, admit:
    infants
    children with definite dyspnoea
    children who look 'toxic'

Box 6.2 *Choice of antibiotic therapy in pneumonia*

NEONATE (< 4 weeks): iv cefotaxime (or benzylpenicillin and gentamicin)

INFANTS AND TODDLERS (< 1 yr): iv co-amoxiclav or iv cefotaxime (or iv flucloxacillin and gentamicin): discuss with paediatric staff

CHILDREN OVER 1 YEAR: oral amoxycillin or erythromycin (if well enough not to require admission)

(Consider erythromycin in school-age child to cover possible *Mycoplasma* infection)

Note: older children with no respiratory difficulty can be treated at home but the GP should be contacted for review.
- *All* children in whom the diagnosis of pneumonia is made should have appropriate antibiotics. The initial choice of drug depends on age (Box 6.2).
- Antibiotics should be given for 7–10 days (except where *Staphylococcus* sp. identified – may need 4–6 weeks).
- Maintenance fluids may be required in those unable to maintain oral intake.
- Oxygen should be administered to keep $Sao_2 > 90\%$; infants preferably via head-box, otherwise by face-mask or nasal cannula; oxygen should be humidified but mist does not help.

Outcome and prognosis

Pneumonia continues to cause a small number of childhood deaths a year in the UK; a wider spectrum of organisms is encountered in children than in adults.

PERTUSSIS AND PERTUSSIS SYNDROME

Background information

- Epidemics of pertussis tend to occur at intervals of 3–4 years, but increased vaccine uptake may change this.
- *Bordetella pertussis* is the causative organism.
- Pertussis is not always prevented by previous immunization.
- It is particularly severe in the first year of life.
- Other organisms (e.g. adenovirus) can produce a similar picture, causing 'pertussis syndrome'.

Diagnostic approach

History

Typical presentation is as follows.

- Coryzal symptoms are followed by an irritant cough within a few days.

- A **paroxysmal cough** develops within 2–3 weeks (incubation period). **Bursts of coughing** (resembling machine-gun fire) *without respiratory pause* are followed by a sudden **whoop** as air is drawn into the lungs.
- **Vomiting, cyanosis, epistaxis** and **seizures** may occur.
- The cough may continue for weeks ('100 day cough').

Examination

The cough is diagnostic (if heard). There may be little or no respiratory distress.

Investigations

- The **FBC** shows absolute lymphocytosis, usually $> 20 \times 10^{-9} \, l^{-1}$.
- **Chest X-ray** shows bronchial wall thickening with small local areas of collapse or consolidation and air trapping.
- **Monitoring of Sa_{O_2}** is essential if there is any history of respiratory distress or apnoea.
- **Pharyngeal or pernasal swabs** (to culture *B. pertussis*) are often taken.
- **Viral culture** and **paired antibody titres** may be helpful.

Management and referral

Little alters the course of the disease, and management is mainly supportive.

- If the child is seen within 2–3 weeks of illness, oral erythromycin should be prescribed for 14 days as it is said to reduce the period of infectivity.
- Avoid provoking factors (e.g. exposure to cold air).
- Beta-2-adrenergic stimulants may reduce paroxysms.
- Cough suppressants rarely have an effect.
- It is reasonable to treat infant siblings with erythromycin.

ACUTE BRONCHITIS

Background information

- Acute bronchitis is the most common cause of acute cough in childhood; it occurs at any age.
- The aetiology is almost always viral.

Diagnostic approach

Typical presentation is as follows:

- Two or three days of **coryzal symptoms** lead to **coughing attacks**.
- There is **little or no pyrexia** and **no respiratory distress or cyanosis**.
- There is **no hyperinflation**.

Investigations

- None usually required.
- **Sputum culture** can be considered in older children to exclude secondary bacterial infection.

Management and referral

- Antibiotics are not needed as almost all attacks are viral; supportive treatment is the rule.
- A cough suppressant (e.g. linctus codeine 5 ml) may assist sleep.
- Admission is rarely needed (unless the social background is poor).

b. COUGH AND WHEEZE IN INFANTS

BACKGROUND INFORMATION

The airways of a baby have a small diameter and wheeze can be a feature of infection and inflammation. This section deals with cough and wheeze presenting in children under 1 year old. Bronchospasm and inflammation, characteristic of asthma, do occur in older infants – thus the differential diagnosis lies largely between a viral lower respiratory tract infection (common in younger babies) and early onset of asthma (in older babies). Rarely an inhaled foreign body or cystic fibrosis may be the cause. Congenital heart disease may present in early infancy with breathlessness and an enlarged liver.

Infants less than 10 months old are likely to have bronchiolitis – viral lower respiratory tract infection (LRTI) – rather than asthma. A plump 10-month-old baby with asthma is easily distinguished from an 8-week-old baby hyperinflated with bronchiolitis, but the conditions do merge.

Bronchiolitis results from viral infection (75% respiratory syncytial virus). The cough, breathlessness and wheeze are often preceded by coryza. There is an annual winter epidemic in the UK which accounts for the hospital admission of 2–3% of all infants.

Asthma occurs rarely under 10 months of age. Wheezing due to asthma may be triggered by viral upper respiratory tract infection (URTI), thus an accurate differential diagnosis often cannot be made at first presentation.

DIAGNOSTIC APPROACH

History

It is important to know the following points:

- **Age** – younger babies will cope less well.
- **Feeding** – expends energy. It is more difficult to coordinate a 'suck, swallow, breathe' pattern if respiration is embarrassed.
- **Previous medical history** – lung disease of prematurity or a history of congenital heart disease may render a baby more susceptible to a severe attack of bronchiolitis.
- **Apnoea** – the baby is at risk and needs observing.
- **Family history** – there may be a past of family history of eczema and asthma.

- **Smoking** – cigarette smoke acts as an irritant and can cause wheezing in susceptible infants. Smoking during pregnancy increases an infant's risk of recurrent wheezy illness.
- **Preceding URTI** may be a feature of either bronchiolitis or asthma.

Examination

Observe the **general demeanour** of the infant (see Chapter 2). In addition, note:

- **Pyrexia** – absent or mild in bronchiolitis and asthma, but significantly raised if either illness is complicated by secondary bacterial infection, e.g. pneumonia (see above).
- **Heart rate** – tachycardia reflects the strain imposed by an increased work of breathing. Hypoxia induces a sympathomimetic response which will also increase heart rate.
- **Colour** – deteriorates with increasing severity of illness and impending respiratory failure.
- **Work of breathing** increases with raised **respiratory rate**. Look for **recession** – manifesting as subcostal recession or paradoxical chest wall movement (diaphragm pulls compliant ribs inwards; intercostal muscles are weak and ribs flexible in infancy), **flaring of nostrils** and a **grunt**. Observe for any prolonged expiratory phase.
- **Effectiveness of breathing** affects **colour**. Note the patient's **degree of hyperinflation** (indicated by a prominent sternum and depressed liver). **Chest auscultation** may reveal widespread wheezes (expiratory more than inspiratory) and fine crepitations (inspiratory more than expiratory) which are characteristic of bronchiolitis. A tight cough and wheeze proceed to moist cough as the disease resolves. Widespread multiphonic wheezes (expiratory more than inspiratory) characterize asthma, but crepitations are unusual.

Investigations

- **Oxygen saturation** is measured to detect significant hypoxia.
- Consider **CXR** – not a routine part of management and usually only indicated when the presentation does not fit the typical pattern.
- **Nasopharyngeal aspirate** – respiratory syncytial virus (RSV) immunofluorescence may identify the usual causative agents in bronchiolitis.

Remember: treatment is more important than investigations

MANAGEMENT AND REFERRAL

Bronchiolitis or asthma

- Give oxygen to correct any hypoxia.
- Age under 6 months – try ipratropium bromide (125–250 µg nebulized) for wheezing. This can be given as four puffs of a 20 µg aerosol via a spacer with face-mask attached.
- Age over 6 months – try a beta-2 adrenoceptor agonist, if the above is not helpful (e.g. salbutamol 1.25–2.5 mg nebulized or four puffs of a 100 µg inhaler via a spacer and face-mask).
- The spacer devices may be used for home management if the baby responds and is only mildly unwell.

Bronchodilators are often not effective in bronchiolitis and are less useful than might be expected in asthma in infants. Only a third show an improvement with nebulized ipratropium after 20 min

- If the infant is hypoxic and **severely unwell**, call for help IMMEDIATELY.
- In asthma follow the flow chart in Figure 6.1.
- Referral guidelines are summarized in Box 6.3.
  Note: Ribavirin – a specific antiviral agent – is sometimes helpful if given early in bronchiolitis. It is nebulized and generally reserved for infants at risk, e.g. those with congenital heart disease (CHD).

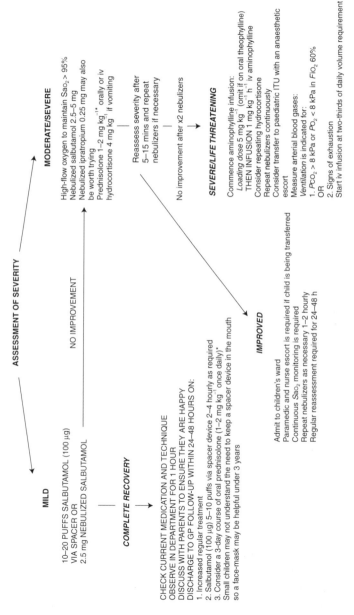

ASSESSMENT OF SEVERITY

MILD

NO IMPROVEMENT

MODERATE/SEVERE

High-flow oxygen to maintain SaO_2 > 95%
Nebulized salbutamol 2.5–5 mg
Nebulized ipratropium 0.25 mg may also
be worth trying
Prednisolone 1–2 mg kg⁻¹* orally or iv
hydrocortisone 4 mg kg⁻¹ if vomiting

Reassess severity after
5–15 mins and repeat
nebulizers if necessary

No improvement after x2 nebulizers

SEVERE/LIFE THREATENING

Commence aminophylline infusion:
Loading dose 5 mg kg⁻¹ (omit if on oral theophylline)
THEN INFUSION 1 mg kg⁻¹ h⁻¹ iv aminophylline
Consider repeating hydrocortisone
Repeat nebulizers continuously
Consider transfer to paediatric ITU with an anaesthetic
escort
Measure arterial blood gases:
Ventilation is indicated for:
1. PCO_2 > 8 kPa or PO_2 < 8 kPa in FiO_2 60%
OR
2. Signs of exhaustion
Start iv infusion at two-thirds of daily volume requirement

10–20 PUFFS SALBUTAMOL (100 μg)
VIA SPACER OR
2.5 mg NEBULIZED SALBUTAMOL

COMPLETE RECOVERY

CHECK CURRENT MEDICATION AND TECHNIQUE
OBSERVE IN DEPARTMENT FOR 1 HOUR
DISCUSS WITH PARENTS TO ENSURE THEY ARE HAPPY
DISCHARGE TO GP FOLLOW-UP WITHIN 24–48 HOURS ON:
1. Increased regular treatment
2. Salbutamol (100 μg) 5–10 puffs via spacer device 2–4 hourly as required
3. Consider a 3-day course of oral prednisolone (1–2 mg kg⁻¹ once daily)*
Small children may not understand the need to keep a spacer device in the mouth
so a face-mask may be helpful under 3 years

IMPROVED

Admit to children's ward
Paramedic and nurse escort is required if child is being transferred
Continuous SaO_2 monitoring is required
Repeat nebulizers as necessary 1–2 hourly
Regular reassessment required for 24–48 h

Fig. 6.1 *Guidelines for management of a child with asthma*

*1997 BTS Guidelines suggest a dose at the lower end of our suggested range, but it is common practice among paediatricians to give a greater dose (at the higher end of the range).

Box 6.3 *Referral guidelines*

REFER FOR ADVICE IF:

the child is moderately or severely unwell (see Chapter 2)

the child is unable to feed

the presentation is unusual – high fever, unilateral signs

apnoea occurs

there is a history of increasing respiratory difficulties and poor colour

the CXR is abnormal

there is more than one attendance in 3 months, refer for long-term managment of a recurrent wheeze

there is a previous history of prematurity or significant illness (e.g. congenital heart disease)

OUTCOME AND PROGNOSIS

- Bronchiolitis usually completely resolves after 2 weeks. Recurrent wheeze in the infant may be a sequel. Deaths rarely occur (and usually only in infants with pre-existing problems). Ventilation is required in 1–2% of infants with bronchiolitis.
- In asthma the long-term outlook is good. Many grow out of the tendency to recurrent wheezing. ONE EPISODE OF WHEEZING DOES NOT CONSTITUTE ASTHMA.

COUGH AND WHEEZE IN CHILDREN AGED 1–16 YEARS

DIFFERENTIAL DIAGNOSIS

1. Asthma (most common).
2. Inhaled foreign body.

3. Less common causes include pneumonia (see above), aspiration and compression by tumours or large vessels (rare).

ASTHMA

Background information

- Asthma is a chronic disease characterized by reversible airway obstruction.
- It is the most common reason for admission of children to hospital in the UK, affecting at least 1 in 10 children.
- Prevalence is apparently rising in the UK.

Diagnostic approach

History

- **Presenting complaints**:
  cough – usually at night or on exercise; it may be the predominant symptom in childhood
  wheeze
  breathlessness
  dyspnoea – difficulty breathing
  trigger factor – (Box 6.4)
- **Previous medical history**: – in cases where the patient has had previous episodes of wheeze it is important to ascertain the following:
  pre-existing lung disease – e.g. bronchopulmonary dysplasia due to prolonged neonatal ventilation
  severity of previous episodes
  previous admissions
- **Current medication** – it is important to know:
  accurate dose
  route
  technique
  effectiveness
- **Previous treatments** – the need for previous courses of steroids should be noted.

Box 6.4 *Trigger factors in asthma*

INFECTION: usually viral (e.g. adenovirus, rhinovirus), typically causing an upper respiratory tract infection

IRRITANTS: e.g. cigarette smoke, aerosols, mist, paint fumes

EXERCISE: especially in cold air

ALLERGENS: e.g. house-dust mite, animal hair or feathers, pollen, food (chocolate, fizzy drinks, tartrazine).

WEATHER: typically a rapid fall in air temperature (e.g. thunderstorm)

EXCITEMENT, EMOTION

- **Allergy**: a tendency to atopy should be noted. There may be a history of hay fever or eczema.
- **Family history**: there may be a family history of asthma, hay fever or eczema.
- **Social history**: the home environment may influence the natural history of asthma, particularly with respect to exposure to cigarette smoke.

Examination

Examination should be directed towards assessment of severity as mild, moderate or severe (see Chapter 3).

- **Basic observations**:
  heart rate may be normal or only slightly raised in mild asthma. A progressive tachycardia suggests increasing severity (see reference tables in Part VI). Bradycardia is a preterminal sign.
  respiratory rate – see below (and table in Part VI).
  temperature – a mild fever (< 38.5 °C) may be present and is usually due to the associated upper respiratory tract infection (e.g. snuffly nose). A higher fever may indicate pneumonia

blood pressure is often not recorded in mild asthma. However, pulsus paradoxus > 20 mmHg indicates severe asthma. Although rarely measured, it is often palpable.

- **Work of breathing:**
  respiratory rate increases with severity but plummets when exhaustion sets in. There is a prolonged expiratory phase
  ability to speak – inability to speak in sentences indicates moderate or severe asthma
  accessory muscles – older children can be seen to use accessory muscles (e.g. sternomastoid) in more severe asthma
  recession – intercostal and/or subcostal recession increase roughly in proportion to severity. This is more obvious in younger children, in whom there is a relatively compliant chest wall

- **Effectiveness of breathing:**
  colour – the patient's colour becomes increasingly pale as severity increases (cyanosis is a late sign)
  hyperexpansion with air trapping and decreased chest excursion is a feature of asthma

- **Auscultation** – the typical auscultatory findings are widespread, expiratory, multiphonic wheezes. However, it is important to note that the degree of wheeze is a poor indicator of severity in asthma. Indeed, a silent chest may indicate severe asthma with hypoventilation (Boxes 6.5 and 6.6).

Box 6.5 *Severe asthma*

Pronounced tachycardia
Pronounced tachypnoea
Pulsus paradoxus > 20 mmHg
SaO_2 < 85%
Peak flow < 50% normal
Markedly increased work of breathing

Box 6.6 *Pre-terminal signs*

Cyanosis
Bradycardia
Exhaustion
Hypotension
Silent chest

Investigations

In the A&E department:

- **Oxygen saturation** (Sao_2) – measurement of saturation should be mandatory in moderate or severe asthma; decreasing Sao_2 indicates severe asthma and an $Sao_2 < 85\%$ in air is *life-threatening*.
- **Peak flow measurement** may be helpful, particularly if the child is over 5 years old and previous values are known. Peak flow values below 50% of expected levels indicate severe asthma, and values below 33% expected are *life-threatening*. (See reference table in Part VI, p. 364.)
- **Chest X-ray** is not a routine investigation in asthma but is indicated in the following situations:
  1. In cases of acute severe asthma which do not respond to the treatment described below. Pneumothorax or lobar collapse should be excluded in these instances.
  2. When an inhaled foreign body cannot be excluded, particularly in a young child.
  3. When chest signs are asymmetrical.
  4. At the first hospital presentation of a moderate or severe episode.
- **Arterial blood gas analysis** is only needed in very severe episodes, usually if mechanical ventilation is considered. Capillary gas samples are acceptable if arterial samples are difficult to obtain. Always call for help!

Management and referral

Management in the A&E department should follow the guidelines in Figure 6.1.

> Respiratory failure in asthma results from exhaustion – it can happen suddenly!
> If concerned, call for help early

Outcome and prognosis

A productive cough is part of the normal recovery phase of asthma, reflecting the increased mucus production which is part of the pathophysiology; it is not an indication for antibiotic therapy. Antibiotics should be prescribed only for specific indications.

With prompt treatment most children will recover well but all should remain on increased medication in the recovery phase. Ideally they should be followed up in asthma clinics.

Long-term management should be directed towards avoidance of trigger factors and discussion of maintenance therapy – a step-by-step guide is published by the British Thoracic Society. Poor control can lead to school absence, psychological problems, chronic chest problems and poor growth.

> **Beware: there are still up to 40–50 child deaths from asthma per year in the UK**

INHALED FOREIGN BODY

Background information

Inhalation of a foreign body typically occurs at age 2–5 years. The precise manifestations depend on the level in the bronchial tree at which the object lodges. These children are in a precarious position as total obstruction can result from movement.

Diagnostic approach

History

- **Onset** is typically sudden without a preceding history of upper respiratory tract infection.
- **Timing** – the incident often happens when the child is active or playing with small objects (e.g. toy, nut) and is unattended.
- **Symptoms** – cough and wheeze are often present, although a laryngeal foreign body may present with stridor (see below).

Examination

Signs are dependent upon the site of the foreign body but may include the following:

- Upper respiratory tree foreign body:
    choking or coughing
    stridor
    cyanosis
    depressed consciousness
- Lower respiratory tree foreign body:
    coughing
    localized rhonchi
    decreased air entry unilaterally
    cyanosis
    depressed conscious level

Investigations

In the collapsed child, investigations take second place to treatment. In a stable child in the A&E department:

1. **Pulse oximetry** - Sao_2 monitoring is mandatory.
2. **Chest X-ray** – films should ideally be taken on inspiration and expiration. Mediastinal shift and localized areas of hyperinflation may only be apparent on expiration and are due to gas trapping distal to the foreign body.
3. **Lateral neck X-ray** may pick up a radio-opaque laryngeal foreign body; other objects may be seen contrasted against laryngotracheal air.
4. **Arterial blood gas** analyses should not be carried out before instigating treatment.

Management

In the A&E department treatment may be given as follows.

Collapsed or unconscious child

The standard 'ABC' approach should be used – see Part III. Emergency tracheostomy may be needed.

Choking

The following techniques may be used to clear the airway if:

the diagnosis is strongly suspected *and/or*

airway opening techniques (head tilt/chin lift and jaw thrust) have failed

- Infants:
  1. Place the baby along one arm in a head-down position (or if the baby is larger, sit down with the baby resting on your thigh). *Up to five blows* are delivered to the back between the scapulae.
  2. If still unrelieved, the baby is turned over and *up to five chest compressions* are given slowly with two fingers, one finger-breadth inferior to the nipple line. Compress to a depth of 1.5–2.5 cm.
- Children: back blows with the spine flexed may be effective in the older child, but the Heimlich manoeuvre can also be used with the child standing or sitting. In the Heimlich manoeuvre a fist is placed against the child's epigastrium. With the other hand placed over the first, both are thrust inwards and upwards ten times (unless the object is expelled before this).

Referral

Always take advice from the attending anaesthetist. Urgent removal of a laryngeal foreign body with a laryngoscope and Magill forceps in the A&E department may be life-saving. Urgent bronchoscopy may be required so that the foreign body can be removed. Occasionally a trans-bronchial approach at thoracotomy will be needed.

Outcome and prognosis

If an inhaled foreign body lodges in the larynx or trachea the outcome is often fatal unless measures are taken to remove it immediately.

c. STRIDOR

BACKGROUND INFORMATION

Stridor is a continuous harsh sound caused by obstruction in the larynx or trachea (i.e. the upper airways). It is predominantly an inspiratory noise, but an expiratory component may be present, especially in lesions involving the subglottic area. There is a higher incidence of stridor in children than in adults, partly because of the anatomical differences. In children:

1. The airways are universally of a smaller size.
2. The larynx is more anterior and superior.
3. The epiglottis is longer and U-shaped.
4. The vocal cords are short and concave.
5. The supporting cartilage of the airways is less well developed and more easily deformed.
6. The airways are more physiologically dynamic owing to higher compliance, so collapse of the trachea can occur during inspiration.

Acute stridor is a frightening symptom for children, parents and doctors. Its causes are listed in Box 6.7.

Box 6.7 *Causes of acute stridor*

Acute laryngotracheobronchitis

Acute epiglottitis or bacterial tracheitis

Foreign body or inhaled hot gases

Acute angioneurotic oedema (anaphylaxis)

Diphtheria

Expanding mediastinal masses

Tetany

Peritonsillar abscess, retropharyngeal abscess

Chronic stridor less commonly presents to the A&E department. However, all cases of chronic stridor can be worsened acutely by any of the above conditions. Causes of chronic stridor include:

laryngomalacia (floppy larynx)
laryngeal web
vocal cord palsy
subglottic haemangioma or stenosis

Problems associated with stridor include airways obstruction, acute hypoxia, feeding problems and (in the chronic cases) failure to thrive.

DIAGNOSTIC APPROACH

History

The following historical factors are important to establish.

- **Age**: foreign body obstruction occurs from approximately 6 months onwards. Acute viral laryngotracheobronchitis (LTB) is common between the ages of 1 year and 3 years. Epiglottitis is most common between the ages of 2 years and 7 years, and bacterial tracheitis is most common under the age of 5 years. Peritonsillar abscess typically occurs in children over 8 years old, whereas retropharyngeal abscess occurs between the ages of 1 year and 3 years.

- **Duration**: viral LTB is usually preceded by coryzal symptoms for 1–2 days, whereas epiglottitis is preceded by dysphagia progressively worsening over a period of hours. Foreign body inhalation usually has sudden onset, although the act of inhalation may be missed.

- **Aggravating or alleviating factors**:
    posture – children with stridor normally assume an upright position and lean forward.
    activity (e.g. feeding)
    agitation – stridor often worsens with agitation
    sleeping – does the stridor persist during sleep?

- **Diurnal variation**: the cough and stridor associated with acute LTB are often worse at night.

- **Associated respiratory noises**:
    1. Cough – a barking cough is typically associated with acute LTB, a 'choking' cough with a foreign body.
    2. Grunt – represents closure of the glottis at the end of the expiration which generates an additional positive end-expiratory

pressure. In many disease states this is necessary to prevent alveoli from collapse. It may be an ominous sign.

- **Current medication**: the patient may be on prescribed or home remedies.
- **Previous medical history**: in particular note a previous history of ventilation or intubation, or of premature delivery. Note any previous admissions with stridor.

Examination

General principles to be applied when assessing a child with stridor:

> The initial examination of a child with acute onset of stridor should consist of observation only
> The aim is **assessment of severity**

1. Do not disturb the child; allow him or her to sit on the carer's lap.
2. Do not leave the child unattended.
3. Do not remove the child from his or her preferred position.
4. Avoid painful or upsetting procedures (e.g. iv access or pharyngeal examination) until experienced personnel and equipment for intubation are available.

- **General appearance**: a child with epiglottitis is typically 'toxic-looking', pale, possibly drooling and shocked; however, a child with bacterial tracheitis may have a similar appearance. A child with acute LTB is typically anxious and lethargic but may appear well, particularly during the daytime. The voice is hoarse and weak in epiglottitis, and hoarse with a barking cough in acute LTB; the child may be aphonic in foreign body aspiration.
- **Basic observations**:
    - **temperature** is typically mildly raised (<38°C) in viral LTB (croup) but may be markedly raised (>38°C) in epiglottitis or bacterial tracheitis
    - **respiratory rate** is often laboured in epiglottis; variable in foreign body aspiration; raised in acute LTB
    - **pulse** is typically raised but may be normal
- **Respiratory system**:
    - **colour** – children with stridor are often pale, but the presence of cyanosis is an urgent and sinister sign

signs of distress – e.g. sternal or subcostal recession
stridor – quality, timing and severity should be recorded
associated respiratory noise – wheezes and coarse crackles
may be associated with acute LTB or tracheitis

Chest auscultation should only be carried out if the child does not become distressed. Try to note:

location of loudest stridor
intensity/asymmetry of breath sounds
other added signs

After this initial assessment, the *severity* of respiratory distress can be assessed (Table 6.2). If the respiratory distress is not severe and the child's condition is stable, the examination can proceed as follows:

tongue and pharynx
tympanic membranes
neck (for masses)
general examination (as described in Chapters 2 and 3)

Table 6.2   *Assessment of severity of respiratory distress in stridor*

Signs	Score 1	Score 2	Score 3	Score 4
1. Colour	Normal ($Sao_2 > 95\%$)	Normal ($Sao_2 > 90\%$)	Normal/pale ($Sao_2 > 85\%$)	Cyanosis ($Sao_2 < 85\%$)
2. Level of consciousness	Normal/alert	Restless when disturbed	Restless at rest	Lethargic
3. Stridor	None	When agitated	Mild at rest	Severe at rest
4. Retraction/recession	None	Mild	Moderate	Severe
5. Air entry	Normal	Mildly reduced	Moderately reduced	Severely reduced (?absent)

Add the score for each factor to obtain the total Stridor Score. As a guide:
mild = score 6 or less
moderate = score 7–8
severe = score 9 or more

At all times the child should be repeatedly reassessed to look for the signs of respiratory failure (Chapter 20).

Investigations

As a general rule investigations should not be undertaken until the initial assessment is complete. All children should have **continuous pulse oximetry**. Patients with severe stridor may require **blood gas analysis**. Other investigations (e.g. **FBC**, **blood cultures**) may be necessary but should be guided by the diagnoses considered.

MANAGEMENT AND REFERRAL

The guidelines below are based on the assessment of respiratory distress in Table 6.2.

- Mild (score 6 or less): child probably does not require admission. Supportive therapy only is required usually but consider treatment as for moderate severity.
- Moderate (score 7–8): consider observations in A&E (possibly with admission to ward, particularly if the child is < 2 yr old); consider a single dose of nebulized budesonide (2 mg) during the period of observation. Some practitioners use an oral dose of steroids.
- Severe (score 9 or greater): call for help. Admission may be required, possibly to an intensive therapy unit (ITU); consider nebulized adrenaline to 'buy time' (see below) if the score is 15+ (very severe). Consider intravenous antibiotics to cover the possibility of bacterial tracheitis (e.g. co-amoxiclav).

OUTCOME AND PROGNOSIS

The outcome varies according to diagnosis, but in general prompt recognition and early intervention will improve the prognosis.

FURTHER READING

British Thoracic Society (1997) *'Step by Step' Guidelines in Asthma.*

7 CHILDREN WITH GASTROINTESTINAL SYMPTOMS

This chapter is divided into four sections:

1. Vomiting
2. Abdominal pain
3. Diarrhoea and vomiting
4. Rectal bleeding

Other symptoms are considered, where relevant, within these sections. For example, constipation is a common symptom in childhood and often presents with rectal bleeding or even 'diarrhoea' (constipation with overflow).

VOMITING

BACKGROUND INFORMATION

Vomiting is a common symptom of illness in children of any age. Management is directed towards:

- Assessing the significance and severity.
- Determining a cause for any persistent vomiting.

> Bile-stained vomit is a significant symptom at any age

The following causes of vomiting need to be considered:

1. Obstruction: e.g. pyloric stenosis, intussusception, appendicitis, volvulus, atresia.
2. Infection: e.g. gastroenteritis, UTI, upper or lower respiratory tract infection.
3. Gastroesophageal reflux.
4. Metabolic: e.g. diabetes, inborn errors of metabolism.

5. Intracranial pathology: e.g. head injury, raised intracranial pressure.
6. Others: e.g. drugs, food intolerance, psychological (in older children).

DIAGNOSTIC APPROACH

History

In addition to a general history the following specific points need to be established, particularly in infants.

- **Age**: the baby with pyloric stenosis typically presents at age 2–8 weeks; intussusception typically occurs at under 2 years (peak 3–9 months).
- **Sex**: pyloric stenosis and intussusception are commoner in boys.
- **Gestation at time of delivery** and **birthweight**: significant vomiting is associated with growth failure if prolonged, allowance being made for prematurity.
- **Feeding pattern since birth** (breast- or bottle-fed, any changes in formula used, etc.).
- **Volume** of milk per feed if bottle-fed and **number** of feeds per day; overfeeding can lead to babies vomiting the 'excess' feed.
- **Whether baby enjoys feed and settles afterwards**.
- **Relationship of vomit to feed**: Does it occur immediately after? Is it spread out through out the intervening hours?
- **Is action of vomiting effortless**? Vomiting should be differentiated from 'posseting', which is the regurgitation of mouthfuls of curdled milk in a young infant.
- **Nature of vomiting**:
    projectile bile-stained vomit suggests a mechanical obstruction
    milk or 'posset'?
    blood – this may indicate oesophagitis and is present in 20% of cases of pyloric stenosis.
- **Family history:** there is a history of pyloric stenosis in about 10% of patients.
- **Weight progress** (vital in assessing the significance of the vomiting).
- **Nature and frequency** of stool:
    loose and frequent, e.g. in gastroenteritis

infrequent, e.g. obstruction

'starvation stools' (small, frequent, green stools, often described by parents as diarrhoea, but characteristic of pyloric stenosis)

bloody stools in intussusception.

- **Any associated symptoms**:

  apparent pain, e.g. screaming and pallor are typical of intussusception

  fever suggests an infective cause

- **Any postural variation that reduces amount of vomit**: an upright posture may help gastro-oesophageal reflux, whereas vomiting associated with winding suggests excessive swallowed air.

Examination

- **Basic observations** – **temperature**, **pulse**, **respiratory rate**, **blood pressure** (will be normal unless the baby is severely unwell).
- **General observations** – is baby **active** and **alert**? Is there evidence of **trauma**?
- Record the **weight** of the baby and plot on appropriate **centile chart**.
- **Fontanelle** – is it sunken, or bulging with distracted suture lines?
- Look for other signs of **dehydration**:

  lax skin with decreased turgor

  dry nappies

  sunken eyes

  dry lips and mucous membranes (see Chaper 21).

- **Ear**, **nose**, **throat** and **mouth** – oral thrush can put babies off feeds.
- **Chest**: if dry and acidotic the respiratory rate will be elevated, perhaps without any other evidence of increased work of breathing. In cases of abdominal distension and/or sepsis in a little baby, the diaphragmatic excursion is limited by space and/or pain, sometimes causing hypoventilation.
- **Circulation**: tachycardia and prolonged capillary refill time will only be present if the baby is very unwell with decreased circulatory volume.
- **Abdomen** – observe for distension or scaphoid abdomen. Visible peristalsis may be seen in pyloric stenosis.

1. **Palpate** all areas for any masses or organomegaly (e.g. a 'full-ness' in the right upper quadrant may be felt in intussusception) and note any evidence of tenderness while palpating. Note the site of abdominal tenderness (see Chapter 7).
2. **Percuss** over any mass to assess its size.
3. **Auscultate** for the presence of normal bowel sounds.
4. Do a **test feed** (see below) to try to assess the swelling of the pylorus in pyloric stenosis.

- A **rectal examination** is important in any baby who is deemed to have significant symptoms. Use smallest finger and check anal ring, tone and the nature and presence of stool (e.g. hard, soft, bloody, in rectum).

If unsure, ask a senior colleague

Test feed

A guide to normal quantities is given in Box 7.1.

1. Position the baby on the carer's lap, the baby's head to the carer's left side.
2. Sit comfortably in front with baby's abdomen exposed, and allow feeding to become established.
3. Gently lay your left hand on the baby's abdomen with index middle and ring fingers in the region of angle between the rectus sheath and liver edge, and palpate gently.
4. The 'olive-sized' pyloric swelling is usually palpable intermittently, as though a wave of peristalsis includes the region of the pylorus but makes the pylorus tight and 'hard' instead of being able to open.

Box 7.1 *Points to remember when assessing feeds*

$30 \text{ ml} = 1 \text{ oz or } 100 \text{ ml} = 3\frac{1}{3} \text{ oz}$

'Normal' neonatal feed intake is approximately 150 ml kg^{-1} (5 oz kg^{-1}) per day

Excessive amounts of feed offered and taken can cause vomiting!

5. If the diagnosis is suspected and a mass is not felt, have a break, inspect for visible peristalsis as stomach fills, and then return to palpation.

6. If the swelling has not been felt and the baby vomits, it is always worth returning to feel again *after* the vomit, as sometimes this is when the mass is most prominent.

7. Always ensure the infant is relaxed and settled.

Investigations

- **Urinalysis** and **microscopy** are essential in all cases.
- Abdominal **ultrasonography** can be used to diagnose pyloric stenosis (but a clinical diagnosis is usually possible by paediatricians).
- **Abdominal X-ray** should be performed if mechanical obstruction is likely (e.g. fluid levels may be seen).
- Other investigations to consider include **septic screen** (see Chapter 5); **stool specimens** (see Chapter 7); further **radiography** (including contrast radiography).

MANAGEMENT AND REFERRAL

- Any baby less than 1 week old with persistent vomiting is likely to have a serious disorder.
- Outside the neonatal period, referral can be judged more on the severity of the illness.
- If the child is only mildly unwell (but thriving) and looks comfortable, reassurance to the carers that the vomiting does not represent a significant problem is required. However, in all cases if unsure refer for advice.

No child should be allowed home with undiagnosed vomiting

OUTCOME AND PROGNOSIS

Most of the conditions mentioned above have an excellent prognosis with appropriate treatment. Notes on most of the important conditions can be found in relevant sections of this book. Short notes follow on some important conditions not specifically covered elsewhere.

Pyloric stenosis

Pyloric stenosis is remedied by a (fairly) simple operation (Ramstedt's procedure), but remember how concerned the parents will be for their small baby. Beware of the phrase 'pyloric tumour', which is easily misinterpreted by carers as implying 'cancer'. Any dehydration needs to be corrected before operation, as there is hyperchloraemic alkalosis.

Gastro-oesophageal reflux

Gastro-oesophageal reflux (GOR) is extremely common and often persists into later infancy. The gastro-oesophageal junction is relatively incompetent in all babies. In some infants food and milk seems to come up as easily as it goes down. If the baby thrives GOR is not a problem apart from the social inconvenience and need for a washing machine. In more severe forms oesophagitis will be present, often causing discomfort before and after feeds. Symptoms suggesting complicated GOR which requires investigation include dysphagia, haematemesis, irritability and failure to thrive.

Paediatric advice is needed and medical treatment including increasing feed thickness, posture of the baby and acid-reducing agents are often effective.

In all but the most severe cases the condition is self-limiting, with the tendency to regurgitate and vomit being much less after the first year of life.

Milk intolerance

True milk intolerance is very rare. Beware changing the milk formula unless it is for a good reason. Knowledge of milk formulae is important.

- The SMA, Cow & Gate, Farley, etc. formulae all contain cow's milk protein; SMA Gold and Cow & Gate Premium are normal first milks.
- The 'hungrier baby' formulae SMA White and C&G Plus are casein-based rather than whey-based; they do not contain any more calories per millilitre but a heavier residue of protein is left in the stomach giving a fuller feeling.

Intussusception

Intussusception is caused by telescoping of the bowel, usually at the ileocaecal region. It causes symptoms of colicky pain and vomiting and if it persists can lead to gangrene secondary to venous obstruction of the intussuscepted bowel and a very unwell child. It is commonest between the ages of 3 months and 12 months but can occur up to the age of about 3 years. Bloodstained mucus per rectum ('red-currant-jelly stool') is classically characteristic of the condition (when advanced) and the child may be shocked.

The typical presentation is of intermittent screaming, pallor and drawing-up of the child's legs. A paucity of abdominal contents is felt in the right iliac fossa and a sausage-shaped fullness (mass) may be present in the right hypochondriac or epigastric region. The diagnosis is suspected on examination supported by plain X-ray (bowel gas pattern) and confirmed by contrast enema which may be used to reduce the intussusception. Surgery is indicated if air/contrast enema fails to reduce the intussusception.

ABDOMINAL PAIN

BACKGROUND INFORMATION

- Abdominal pain in childhood can be recurrent or acute.
- Recurrent abdominal pain affects 10% of schoolchildren and is generally a less urgent problem than acute abdominal pain. It can be defined as three episodes of abdominal pain in a 3-month period,

Table 7.1 *Common causes of acute abdominal pain by age*

	Surgical	Medical*
Infancy		
Relatively common	Strangulated hernia Intussusception Midgut volvulus	Urinary tract infection Pneumonia
Less common	Appendicitis Testicular torsion	Cow's milk protein/lactose intolerance Non-accidental injury
Rare	Complications of Meckel's diverticulitis Hirschsprung's disease or other intestinal obstruction	Lead poisoning Porphyria
Childhood		
Relatively common	Appendicitis Trauma (bowel, pancreas, spleen)	Psychological, abdominal migraine Mesenteric adenitis Urinary tract infection Respiratory tract infection (e.g. tonsillitis, pneumonia) Constipation Infectious mononucleus
Less common	Testicular torsion	Hepatitis Haemolytic uraemic syndrome Henoch–Schönlein purpura Diabetes mellitus Sickle-cell crisis
Rare	Complications of Meckel's diverticulitis	Pancreatitis Peptic ulcer Ulcerative colitis

* Medical causes account for 90% of cases.

interfering with regular activities. It is less likely to present to the A&E department. The children generally look well and investigation, if indicated, should be directed by the general practitioner who is better placed to know the family background.

- Acute abdominal pain is more likely to present to A&E. It can be difficult to assess, especially in a young infant. Both medical and surgical conditions have to be considered; a list of possibilities is given in Table 7.1. Most hospital admissions for abdominal pain result from acute appendicitis or non-specific abdominal pain (NSAP), including mesenteric adenitis. The term 'NSAP' is applied to children whose presentation is similar to acute appendicitis, but whose pain is more diffuse and unaccompanied by peritonism or guarding.
- Adolescents: the causes of abdominal pain are the same as for younger children, but remember:
  1. Certain conditions are more common, e.g. torsion, infectious mononucleosis.
  2. Gynaecological causes need to be considered in an adolescent girl (e.g. menstruation, pelvic inflammatory disease, ovarian cyst, ectopic pregnancy).

DIAGNOSTIC APPROACH

History

A detailed history is required, and reference should be made to Chapters 2 and 3 describing the assessment of the unwell child and infant. The following points should be specifically recorded when assessing an infant or child presenting with abdominal pain.

Presenting complaint

Nature of the pain
- **Localization**: the older child should be asked to describe the pain; the pre-school child will often point to the painful area on request. In infants crying and irritability may be the only signs of pain. A dull ache or sharp pain in the suprapubic region usually comes from the bladder.

- **Severity**: very difficult to elicit in pre-school children, but older children may be able to guide you. Questions such as 'What do you do when you get the pain?' and 'Does the pain make you cry?' may be helpful in pre-school children. Infants pose a problem, but it may be useful to ask the carer if the infant can be distracted with toys.
- **Periodicity**: the older child and even the pre-school child should be able to indicate, with the help of parents, whether the pain is **persistent** or **colicky**. Carers may observe patterns of pain in their infants.
  1. Intermittent or colicky pain usually relates to distension or paralysis of bowel, ureter or bile duct. Conditions such as intussusception, gastroenteritis or evening colic in babies may present in this fashion.
  2. Persistent pain in the lower abdomen is typical of NSAP, appendicitis or urinary tract infection; persistent pain in the upper abdomen is typical of pneumonia or gastritis.

Precipitating factors

In older children the pain of peptic ulceration may be precipitated by food. In an infant any **relationship of pain to feeding** should be sought, as it may suggest GOR.

Associated symptoms

- **Vomiting** is present in the majority of cases of abdominal pain in infancy; it is an imprecise pointer to organic causes in older children. It may be an early feature (and is often bilestained) in intussusception or in other causes of bowel obstruction. The assessment of a vomiting child is considered in the preceding section.
- **Diarrhoea**: what parents (or children) mean by this term should be carefully established (see below). The association of diarrhoea with abdominal pain is highly suggestive of gastroenteritis but may occasionally occur as a response to systemic infection (e.g. pneumonia, otitis media, pelvic appendicitis, intussusception or Hirschsprung's disease). **Bloody diarrhoea** may be a feature of some infective causes, or of intussusception, colitis or haemolytic uraemic syndrome.
- **Fever**: low-grade fever (< 38°C) is associated with appendicitis but

fever may be high (> 38.5°C) in UTI, pneumonia or other severe systemic infections.

- **Specific symptoms** for example:
  cough suggesting pneumonia
  dysuria suggesting UTI in an older child (if urethral); suprapubic dysuria may indicate pelvic appendicitis
  rash suggesting Henoch-Schönlein purpura
  sore throat suggesting tonsillitis or mesenteric adenitis
  jaundice suggesting hepatic causes

Examination

See Chapters 2 and 3. Infants and children should be assessed opportunistically but systematically.

Basic observations, including **blood pressure**, should be recorded for all children with abdominal pain. The **state of hydration** must be assessed, and evidence of **shock** sought (see Chapter 21).

Because of the multitude of possible causes a full examination should be carried out. Pneumonia may be missed if chest examination is omitted, or tonsillitis if the ENT examination is neglected.

The following details relate to the examination findings in the abdomen.

Inspection

The abdomen of the infant and toddler is usually protuberant in the upright posture; even experienced paediatricians have difficulty distinguishing a normal 'pot belly' from a pathological one.

- **Abdominal distension** could be caused by:
  fat
  fluid
  faeces   } percussion may help to distinguish
  flatus
  visceromegaly
  muscle hypotonia
  exaggerated lordosis

faeces suggests constipation; **flatus** suggests air swallowing, mal-absorption or possibly intestinal obstruction; **fluid** suggests ascites (e.g. nephrotic syndrome).

- Respiration is usually abdominal in type in children up to school age.
- Small umbilical hernias and hydroceles are a frequent finding and slight separation (divarication) of the rectus muscle is normal.
- Visible loops of bowel are sometimes noted in malnourished infants, but **visible peristalsis** of the stomach may be a sign of pyloric stenosis.

Palpation

- A calm and careful palpation of the abdomen, including **hernial orifices** and the **external genitalia**, should be carried out. The abdomen should be palpated in **quadrants**, with the examiner starting furthest away from the obvious site of pain if possible.
- Try to avoid making the child cry; occasionally you may have to palpate the abdomen with the infant crawling or standing.
- The toddler or pre-school child who resists abdominal examination may be coaxed by distraction techniques. If these fail, use the child's hand to guide yours around the abdomen – a fretful child may allow you to assess abdominal tenderness in this fashion.
- A useful technique for assessing abdominal tenderness in a 'jumpy' older child is to palpate with a stethoscope. If in doubt as to the significance of the tenderness, say 'I'm just going to listen with my stethoscope', gradually increasing the pressure as you do so – often quite firm pressure can be tolerated where previously there was 'tenderness'. Light percussion in the quadrants may also help in localization.
- Note that the spleen and liver may be palpable in infants and small children, and rarely normal kidneys. Abnormal **masses** may be felt (e.g. a sausage-shaped mass in the right hypochondrium in intus-susception).
- The **site of the greatest tenderness** may give an indication to diagnosis (e.g. right iliac fossa in appendicitis, left iliac fossa in constipation, flank in pylonephritis).
- As a general guide, the further the pain is from the umbilicus the more likely it is to be organic. Unilateral pain is also likely to be significant.

Note: 'Rebound' tenderness, as described in some surgical texts, should never be elicited.

Auscultation

The technique described above may be useful in determining tenderness, and the presence or absence and type (e.g. 'tinkling' in obstructive causes or silent in ileus) of bowel sounds may be a diagnostic pointer in establishing causes of abdominal pain.

Rectal examination

Rectal examination should *not* be routine in children; always explain before you do it, and use your 'little finger for little children' and index finger for older children. Examine for:

   masses (faeces, polyps)

   local abdominal or pelvic tenderness (e.g. appendicitis, especially pelvic)

   blood or other staining.

Examination of genitalia

The scrotum may be swollen in Henoch–Schönlein purpura and idiopathic scrotal oedema, but if the testicle is painful, swollen, tender or red the most important diagnosis to consider is testicular torsion.

   Note that bacterial epididymo-orchitis is rare in childhood unless there is an underlying renal abnormality, but presumed viral episodes can occur.

Investigations

Where the cause is not obvious the following are indicated as A&E investigations:

- **Full blood count**: often non-specific because neutrophilia is often found in urinary tract infection or acute appendicitis. Sickle screen may be indicated in certain circumstances.
- **Blood biochemistry** may be indicated in certain circumstances, including **glucose** (as diabetes may present with acute abdominal

pain) and **amylase** (to exclude rare cases of pancreatitis), for example.

- **Blood culture** may be indicated as part of a septic screen (see Chapter 5) in possible infective causes.
- **Urine microscopy** and **culture** (and **dipstick analysis** for protein and glucose) should be routine.
- **Radiography**: erect and supine X-rays of the abdomen may show signs of intestinal obstruction or intussusception (see above); ultrasound examination is occasionally helpful in confirming the latter and possible cases of renal colic. Chest X-ray may show signs of lower lobe pneumonia.

MANAGEMENT AND REFERRAL

The medical and surgical management of the child with acute abdominal pain depends on the underlying diagnosis. However, adequate attention must be paid to resuscitation of the patient (see Part III) with fluid replacement, which is equally important prior to surgery. Adequate provision should be made for suitable analgesia (see Chapter 25). An obvious surgical cause is an indication for referral to a surgeon with training in paediatric surgery. Unless a surgical cause is obvious, refer any child in whom there is diagnostic doubt to a senior paediatrician. A judicious period of observation may be helpful and in general greater caution is advised the younger the child. See also the notes on individual conditions below.

OUTCOME AND PROGNOSIS

The outcome and prognosis depend upon the individual diagnosis.

SPECIFIC CONDITIONS

Acute appendicitis

Typically the pain of acute appendicitis moves from the central abdomen to the right iliac fossa. It is associated with vomiting (usually after the pain) and anorexia. Diarrhoea may occur in a pelvic appendicitis. There is often a raised temperature and pulse and a low-grade fever; localized tenderness may be associated with peritonism and guarding.

Beware this condition in the pre-school child as the clinical course may be modified, particularly if antibiotics have been administered for a presumed respiratory infection. Late presentation (following perforation) often occurs in the younger child.

Note that investigations are less important in making a decision to operate than repeated clinical assessment, as a full blood count or radiography are not helpful in differentiating from other causes of abdominal pain.

Non-specific abdominal pain

Non-specific abdominal pain (NSAP) is a term applied to children whose presentation is similar to acute appendicitis, but the pain is more diffuse and unaccompanied by signs of peritonism or guarding. Children with mesenteric adenitis are included in this group, but the latter diagnosis can really only be made on finding enlarged mesenteric lymph nodes at operation and a normal appendix. The condition usually settles over 24–48 h without any specific treatment, but admission to hospital is needed occasionally because of diagnostic difficulty.

Constipation

Constipation is a common condition presenting to A&E departments, usually as acute abdominal pain but occasionally as rectal bleeding or 'diarrhoea' (overflow). The history may be helpful, but palpation of a loaded descending colon and a rectum full of faeces make the diagnosis; X-rays are not required routinely. Bleeding can be caused by an anal fissure, and fear of evacuation (secondary to an anal tear) may cause the constipation in young children. Hirschsprung's disease should be considered in any child in whom the history is of 'always' being constipated with poor growth, particularly if there was late passage of meconium and usual treatments are ineffective.

Treatment of constipation may involve softeners (e.g. lactulose), stimulants (e.g. bisacodyl) or enemas (e.g. Micralax). Advice about diet (e.g. increased fluid and high-fibre intake) should be given and follow-up arranged with the GP. Occasionally inpatient admission will be required.

Acute obstruction

- Acute obstruction may be congenital (e.g. bowel atresias, volvulus due to malrotation, or Hirschsprung's disease) or acquired (e.g. strangulated inguinal hernia, adhesions). Vomiting is an early feature of intussusception but obstruction is a late complication.
- The clinical signs include abdominal pain and signs of peritonitis, distension, absent or high-pitched bowel sounds and bile-stained or faeculent vomiting.
- Investigations in the A&E department should include plain abdominal X-ray (which may show loops of distended bowel and possible fluid levels) and venepuncture (blood count, electrolytes – which may need correction – and blood culture).
- Management principles:
  1. Delay surgery to resuscitate fully.
  2. Pass a nasogastric tube and allow free drainage with intermittent aspiration.
  3. Correct shock with iv fluid and give enough to cover maintenance and losses.
  4. Refer for surgical assessment early.

Others

Other conditions causing abdominal pain include:

> UTI (see Chapter 8)
> intussusception (see above)
> diabetes mellitus (see Chapter 21)
> respiratory tract infections (see Chapter 6).

ACUTE DIARRHOEA AND VOMITING

BACKGROUND INFORMATION

Diarrhoea may be considered as altered *consistency* or *frequency* of stool. It should be borne in mind that infants do not usually have formed stools and a breast-fed baby may pass a stool following each feed;

therefore you need to assess normal pattern for that child and note any *alterations*.

> **The most important problem in acute gastroenteritis is that of DEHYDRATION**

Acute diarrhoea and vomiting (D&V) may result from toxic or infective insult. Infective gastroenteritis may be:

- Viral:
    rotavirus (the commonest single infective agent in UK); usually occurs as seasonal outbreaks (December to February)
    enteric adenovirus (5%)
    small round viruses
    Norwalk virus (10%)
- Bacterial:
    Campylobacter jejuni (6% – the commonest *invasive* pathogen in the UK)
    Shigella (1%)
    Salmonella (2%)
    E. coli
    Vibrio cholerae
    Yersinia enterocolitica
- Parasitic:
    Giardia lamblia
    Cryptosporidium (*Entamoeba histolytica*)
- Other causes of acute diarrhoea are shown in Box 7.2.

Box 7.2 *Uncommon causes of acute diarrhoea*

Meningitis
UTI
Diabetic ketoacidosis
Acute appendicitis
Intussusception
Hirschsprung's enterocolitis
Others (pyloric stenosis, otitis media)

DIAGNOSTIC APPROACH

History

- A **prodomal illness** is unlikely but the diarrhoea may be associated with viral infection (URTI symptoms).
- **Vomiting** may *precede* diarrhoea by up to 48 h.
- **Abdominal cramps**.
- **Watery stools** and/or **bloody mucus stools** (the latter suggests invasive organisms but consider intussusception).

Examination

The diagnosis is easier to make when diarrhoea *and* vomiting are apparent; vomiting alone is more worrying and requires careful assessment to exclude other systemic illnesses (see Chapter 7). The younger the child, the more care is required in making the diagnosis.

- **General observations**:

    Is the child **mildly, moderately or severely unwell** (see Chapters 2 and 3)?

    Is the child **feeding/drinking well**?

    Is there **vomiting**? **How much**? (see p. 62)

    Is the child **thirsty**? (but note that if a baby is very dehydrated it may not be interested in fluids).

    Is there evidence of **decreased urine output**? (e.g. fewer than four wet nappies in 24 h or a dry overnight nappy is an indicator of dehydration).

- **Basic observations**:

    temperature: a mild pyrexia is usual, tending to be higher with invasive organisms (*Campylobacter*, *Shigella*, certain *E. coli* strains)

    pulse: typically raised, particularly with pyrexia and increasing dehydration

    blood pressure: preserved until severe dehydration/shock

- **Assessment of clinical degree of dehydration**:

    1.   MILD (< 5%) – not unwell, dry mucous membranes, thirsty.

2. MODERATE (5–10%) – lethargic, sunken fontanelle and eyes, decreased skin turgor, oliguria, maybe tachycardia/tachypnoea.
3. SEVERE (> 10%) – shocked (see Chapter 21), hypotension, peripheral shutdown; plus all the above features.

- Beware certain pitfalls:

    Watery diarrhoea may be mistaken for urine output in nappies.

    Mouth-breathing babies are always 'dry-mouthed'.

    Thin babies and children can cause difficulty in assessing skin turgor – use several sites.

    Crying increases pressure and makes a sunken fontenelle appear normal (examine the baby when not crying if at all possible).

Investigations

In mild cases no investigations are necessary. In other cases the following tests may be helpful:

- **Weight** – accurate weighing is critical for calculating fluid requirements and assessing success of rehydration.
- **U&E**, **creatinine**, **glucose** – required in moderate or severe cases.
- **Stool** – microscopy, culture and sensitivity, ELISA may be required if there is blood or mucus in the stool which may indicate *Shigella*, *Campylobacter* or *Salmonella* infection.
- **FBC** and **haematocrit** (in moderate to severe cases, or when the diagnosis is uncertain).
- Consider:

    urinary urea, creatinine and sodium measurement in incipient renal failure

    urine, blood and CSF culture if systemic sepsis is suspected, especially in an infant

    abdominal X-ray if abdomen is distended or tender

MANAGEMENT AND REFERRAL

Mild to moderate dehydration

- Oral rehydration is appropriate in mild cases and 90% of cases of moderate dehydration.

Breast-feeding should be continued uninterrupted.

- Use of oral rehydration solutions (e.g. Dioralyte, Rehidrat or Electrolade) at a rate of 150 ml kg^{-1} per day is appropriate. Additional water (or breast milk) is given to satisfy thirst.
- The total volume should be given as frequent small feeds and should not be prolonged beyond 48 h without milk supplementation.
- There is no reason to use regrading (quarter strength, half strength, etc.) on reintroduction of milk as there is no evidence that it has any effect on development of lactose intolerance, but the practice is still followed for infants under 6–9 months (without good reason as transient diarrhoea returns in 80% on reintroduction of milk).
- Antidiarrhoeal agents should be avoided and antibiotics are not usually indicated except in specific circumstances (e.g. metronidazole for giardiasis).
- Antibiotics are not indicated unless there is evidence of systemic infection. If they are considered, discuss with senior A&E or paediatric staff.
- Arrange for review of the child by medical staff (GP or A&E) if symptoms persist over 48 h (or change at all); warn parents that gastroenteritis lasts up to 7 days and give advice sheet, if available.

  Note: the most frequent concern of parents is the worry about oral dehydration in the presence of vomiting. Calculate the time interval between oral fluids and vomiting – if greater than a few minutes much of the fluid will be absorbed. Smaller amounts of fluids are usually the key to preventing vomiting; oral rehydration should be continued.

In moderate to severe dehydration

- Children must be referred for consideration of iv rehydration.
- Take blood samples (as indicated above) while obtaining intravenous access.
- If the patient is in shock, manage as per the protocol outlined in Chapter 21 (i.e. 20 ml kg^{-1} fluid and reassess).
- In all other cases, calculate the fluid deficit to be replaced, as follows:

> percentage dehydration × weight (in kg) × 10
> (i.e. 10 kg infant 7.5% dehydrated needs 750 ml replacement)

- In addition normal maintenance fluids need to be calculated (see Appendix 2) and added to the deficit volume, and the total given over 24 h.
- Until electrolytes are known, the usual fluid to commence rehydration with is 'dextrose saline' (sodium chloride 0.18% and glucose 0.4%).

  Note:
  1. If the serum sodium ion concentration is known to be less than 130 mmol l^{-1}, replacement and maintenance should be with 0.45% sodium chloride and 5% glucose solution.
  2. In the rarer situation of a high Na^+ concentration, losses should be replaced using the 0.45% NaCl 4% solution also but calculated over 48 h. Maintenance fluids should be given at two-thirds the normal rate until $Na^+ < 150$ mmol l^{-1}. This avoids sudden falls in sodium concentration, which may cause fits.

- Severe acidosis (plasma bicarbonate < 12 mmol l^{-1} or pH < 7.0) can be treated by providing approximately half the calculated deficit of bicarbonate once fluid resuscitation is in progress:

  deficit (mmol) = weight (kg) × 0.3 × base deficit

- It is not usually necessary to add potassium chloride to infusion fluids usually until the potassium concentration is known, or urine is flowing; it should then be added at 3 mmol kg^{-1} per 24 h. Remember that total body potassium may be depleted with a normal serum concentration.

OUTCOME AND PROGNOSIS

- Mortality from acute gastroenteritis is < 1% in severe hospital cases in the UK.
- Secondary food intolerance is relatively common (5%).
- Temporary 'regrading failure' occurs in approximately 20% and has been termed the 'post-enteritis syndrome' in which there is

temporary failure to tolerate lactose, or cow's-milk protein intolerance. Persistent diarrhoea (> 2 weeks) should be referred.
- The long-term prognosis for the majority of properly managed patients in the developed world is excellent.

RECTAL BLEEDING

BACKGROUND INFORMATION

- The passage of small amounts of blood per rectum in childhood is surprisingly common and is rarely of sinister significance.
- The commonest causes are a simple anal fissure (associated with constipation) or self-limiting infective colitis (Box 7.3)

Box 7.3 *Causes of rectal bleeding*

Anal fissure
Infective colitis (*Shigella, Salmonella, Campylobacter*)
Inflammatory bowel disease
Juvenile polyps (usually rectal)
Meckel's diverticulum
Intussusception
Bleeding disorders
Henoch–Schönlein purpura
Haemolytic uraemic syndrome
Rectal prolapse
Upper gastrointestinal bleeding
Sexual abuse

DIAGNOSTIC APPROACH

History

Follow the procedures outlined in Part I and in this chapter. Specific enquiry should be made regarding the following:

- **Length of history**: acute onset may suggest an infective cause but long-standing bleeding may indicate an intestinal disorder (e.g. polyps or inflammatory bowel disease).
- **Amount of bleeding**: small amounts of blood are passed with the motion in a constipated child, but significant haemorrhage may occur in a bleeding disorder.
- **Nature of the bleeding**: lower GI bleeding causes bright-red bleeding that is passed around or mingled with the stool. Upper GI bleeding results in altered blood or melaenic stools.
- **Pain**: usually indicates a fissure.
- **Associated symptoms**:
     diarrhoea suggests infective causes
     hard, infrequent motions suggest constipation and anal tearing, with perianal pain on defaecation
     mucus per rectum suggests inflammatory bowel disease or a polyp
     abdominal pain may be due to infective colitis but, particularly if severe, should arouse suspicion of conditions such as intussusception.
- **Family history**: e.g. a family history of polyposis coli may be significant.

Examination

A general guide to the examination of the unwell child is found in Chapter 3 and examination of the abdomen is considered earlier in this chapter.

- Clues in the general examination may be obtained by specific findings – for example, the presence of skin changes in Henoch–Schönlein purpura (HSP), or arthritis in HSP or inflammatory bowel disease.

- Attention should be paid to adequate visualization of the perianal region. A paediatric proctoscope may be helpful.
- Direct visualization of the stool should be accompanied by testing for occult blood as necessary, although false positives may be obtained in a child receiving vitamin C supplements.

Investigations

Investigation will depend upon the urgency of the clinical presentation. For example, intussusception may present as a shocked infant in need of fluid resuscitation and **urgent radiography** (see p. 67). In contrast, a constipated child may require no investigation, and in cases of bloody diarrhoea a **stool culture** may be all that is required. Other investigations that may be helpful include **FBC**, **ESR**, **ferritin**, **serum electrolytes**, **clotting studies**. Referral for investigations such as colonoscopy may be rarely required.

MANAGEMENT AND REFERRAL

- Management is according to the underlying condition.
- The commonest cause is constipation, which can be treated with increased fluid intake, stool softeners (e.g. lactulose as an osmotic laxative), stimulant laxatives (e.g. bisacodyl) and enemas (e.g. Micralax Micro-enema), either singly or in combination. These are short-term measures and adequate attention should be paid to bowel retraining and the introduction of adequate fluid, fibre and fruit into the diet. Longer-term follow-up should be arranged with the GP to assess the underlying causes. Note that occasional cases of severe constipation will present with 'diarrhoea' (overflow).
- Infective diarrhoea is managed according to the principles outlined on pages 76–81.
- Other cases should be referred for paediatric assessment and follow-up.

OUTCOME AND PROGNOSIS

The prognosis depends on the cause, but the symptom does not carry a sinister prognosis in the majority of cases.

8 CHILDREN WITH URINARY SYMPTOMS

This chapter concentrates on common presentations only. Dysuria is an obvious urinary symptom but this section of the book also brings together other presentations of urinary tract infection in childhood. Haematuria is dramatic and frightening if gross but it is also a frequent incidental finding on routine testing. Oedema has many causes and these are discussed here for convenience, although nephrotic syndrome is the important renal cause to exclude.

DYSURIA

BACKGROUND INFORMATION

- By far the most important diagnosis to exclude in a child presenting with dysuria is urinary tract infection (UTI) which is common in both infants and children.
- Younger children with UTI may present with less specific symptoms. They often do not complain of 'dysuria', discomfort being inferred from other behaviour.
- Factors that predispose to UTI include incomplete emptying of the bladder, constipation, poor fluid intake, vesicoureteric reflux and renal tract abnormalities.
- It is essential to establish an accurate diagnosis of urinary tract infection before starting treatment and commencing investigations to exclude an underlying abnormality.
- Most infections are caused by normal bowel commensals (> 90% of first infections are attributable to *E. coli*).
- In the neonatal period, infection may be haematogenously acquired and bacteraemia is present in > 60% of cases.
- Veiscoureteric reflux of infected urine causes renal cortical scarring, especially in infants. It is responsible for up to 20% of all cases of

chronic renal failure (CRF) in children and is a significant cause of end-stage renal failure in young adults.
- The younger the child the greater is the risk of renal damage from infection (especially if vesicoureteric reflux is present).
- In the neonatal period UTI is twice as common in boys but in older children it is more common in girls (1–2% in schoolgirls, 0.2% in schoolboys).
- The differential diagnosis of dysuria includes candidiasis or other causes of vulvitis or balanitis, irritation by underwear, soaps or bubble baths, and trauma or sexual abuse.
- In view of these implications, it is important that UTI is *proved* by urine culture and that the child is not just treated on the basis of symptoms.

DIAGNOSTIC APPROACH

History

Neonatal period (< 1 month)

- **Irritability, refusal to feed, vomiting, failure to thrive, prolonged jaundice, diarrhoea**.
- If *septicaemic* the baby will normally be febrile and severely unwell: the condition may mimic meningitis.

Pre-school child

- **Diarrhoea and vomiting, poor weight gain, fever, malaise, frequency, dysuria, enuresis, haematuria, loin pain** (rare).
- If *septicaemic* (especially if < 1 year) the child may look febrile and severely unwell, raising the possibility of meningitis.

Older children

- **Dysuria, haematuria, incontinence, urgency, frequency**. Very few have **loin pain** and **pyrexia** suggesting pyelonephritis.

Examination

Examination should follow the guidelines in Chapters 2 and 3, but particular note should be made of the **blood pressure** and **palpation of abdomen** (for **kidneys** and **bladder**).

Investigations

In the A&E department the following investigations should be carried out.

- **Urine** for microscopy, culture and sensitivities. Note that the reliability of results must be weighed against methods of collection:
    older children – a mid-stream urine (MSU) specimen should be collected (ideally two)
    young child/infant – ideally a clean catch (two) or suprapubic aspirate should be obtained
In most units, it is normal policy to send the sample for urgent microscopy: pyuria suggests infection but it can occur as a response to fever. A finding of 50–100 white cells or more per ml of urine on microscopy is often taken to indicate infection prior to the results of culture.
Note: traditional dipstick testing can be unreliable but several units use the technique for three factors: leucocyte esterase, nitrite and protein. A sample *negative* for all three is considered free from infection although some paediatric nephrologists consider that the risk of an underlying renal abnormality harbouring organisms that do not produce nitrite is greater below the age of 2 years. Consequently it is recommended that urine microscopy is performed in this age group.
- **Full blood count** in a moderately or severely unwell child.
- **Blood cultures** are required for the neonate, young infant or toxic child.
- **Urea**, **electrolytes**, **creatinine** testing in a dehydrated or severely unwell infant or child, or those with pre-existing renal problems.

Note: Since UTI enters the differential diagnosis of a febrile child a full **septic screen** may be required.

MANAGEMENT AND REFERRAL

- Once the urine specimen is collected, start **antibiotics** if UTI is suspected. Give the antibiotics intravenously if:

  the child is vomiting

  the child is toxic

  when the diagnosis is uncertain but potentially serious, as in neonates

  In other cases oral antibiotics can be prescribed, the usual choice being trimethoprim (4 mg kg^{-1} twice daily). Alternatives include co-amoxiclav and the cephalosporins.
- Other therapeutic measures include a **high fluid intake** and **antipyretic treatment**.

Further investigations

All children with a proven UTI should be referred to a paediatrician for follow-up and further investigation. As a general guide:

- *Children aged < 1 year* require ultrasound and dimercaptosuccinic acid (DMSA) scans to detect renal scars, and a micturating cystourethrogram (MCUG) to detect vesicouretic reflux.
- *Children aged 1–5 years* require ultrasound and DMSA scans but a MCUG only if scars are detected or if there is a history of recurrent UTI.
- *Children aged over 5 years* require only an ultrasound scan of the kidney unless abnormalities are detected.

All children should receive prophylactic antibiotics at night (for example, trimethoprim 2 mg kg^{-1} at night) until investigations are complete, and this should be advised in a letter from the A&E department.

Note: A DMSA scan is not carried out until 6 weeks after UTI. The child can be referred to a general or renal paediatrician directly or through the general practitioner.

OUTCOME AND PROGNOSIS

After the first UTI:

> 60% have normal kidneys
> up to 30% have vesicoureteric reflux (although this has been found in normal children under 5 years old)
> 10% show scarring from vesicoureteric reflux
> 7% show obstructon (anatomical or neurogenic)
> 3% show duplex or horseshoe kidneys

HAEMATURIA

BACKGROUND INFORMATION

- Macroscopic (visible) haematuria is a symptom that usually results in children being brought to the doctor promptly and is a cause of understandable concern to parents. Microscopic haematuria is more frequent than gross haematuria but only a small quantity of blood (1 ml of blood in 1000 ml urine) is necessary to make the urine appear red.
- In most cases, minimal investigation will be required and the source of blood may be anywhere from glomerulus to urethra, but most cases in childhood are due to a primary glomerular cause.
- It is important to remember that a number of substances can turn the urine red (Box 8.1). These need to be excluded before a true haematuria is said to be present.

Box 8.1 *Causes of red urine*

HAEMPOSITIVE (dipstick positive)
- Haemoglobinuria
- Myoglobinuria

HAEMNEGATIVE (dipstick negative)
- Metabolites
    Homogentisic acid
    Porphyrin
    Melanin
- Drugs
    Salicylates
    Iron sorbitol
    Nitrofurantoin
    Methyldopa
    Levodopa
    Metronidazole
    Chloroquine
- Foods (e.g. beetroot)

- Blood in the urine is identified most readily by a 'dipstick' (reagent strips such as Haematest or Labstix), using a peroxidase that reacts with haemoblobin; greater than 1+ is considered positive. The dipstick tests for haemoglobin, not red blood cells (RBCs). Any chemical that reacts with the peroxidase will produce a positive test, so all positive dipstick screens must be confirmed by *urine microscopy* to confirm the presence of RBCs. On urine microscopy > 5 erythrocytes per mm^3 of urine is usually considered significant.
- The prevalence of isolated microscopic haematuria in children and adolescents is approximately 1.5% in population statistics, the majority of children being asymptomatic and never developing significant renal disease. Up to 3% of normal schoolchildren will be positive on one occasion and 1% on two or more occasions.
- A fuller list of causes appears in Table 8.1.

Table 8.1 *Causes of haematuria*

Glomerular	Non-glomerular
Inherited	Congenital tubulointerstitial
Alport's syndrome	(vesicoureteric)
Familial benign haematuria	Renal cystic disease
Acquired	Inherited metabolic disorder
IgA nephropathy	Acquired tubulointerstitial (vesicoureteric)
Glomerulonephritis	Allograft rejection
Minimal change disease	Nephrotoxic drugs
Systemic	Analgesic abuse
Systemic lupus erythematosus	Radiation
Henoch–Schönlein purpura	Vesicoureteric reflux
Haemolytic-uraemic syndrome	Idiopathic
Goodpasture's syndrome	Urinary tract disorders
Amyloidosis	Urolithiasis
Diabetic nephropathy	Hypercalciuria
Infectious	Tumours
Post-streptococcal	Vascular abnormalities
(glomerulonephritis)	Trauma
Subacute bacterial endocarditis	Obstruction
Shunt nephritis	Haemorrhagic cystitis
Hepatitis	Infection
Malaria, toxoplasmosis	Other (idiopathic urethrorrhagia)

DIAGNOSTIC APPROACH

History

Age

The importance of age as a factor is illustrated in Table 8.2, which differentiates the common causes of haematuria in different groups.

Table 8.2 *Causes of haematuria in different age groups*

Newborn and infant (< 1 year)	Pre-school age (1–5 years)	School age and adolescent (> 5 years)
Trauma (catheterization)	Infection	Infection
Ischaemic renal injury	Renal malformation	Menstruation
Coagulopathy (including renal vein thrombosis)	Glomerulonephritis	Trauma
	Trauma	Glomerulonephritis
Renal malformation		

Pattern

The pattern of the episodes of haematuria is important. For example, persistent microscopic haematuria with recurrent episodes of gross haematuria, particularly if the episodes are associated with viral illness, suggests IgA nephropathy. The same pattern associated with dysuria and back (or flank) pain suggests urinary tract infection, hypercalcaemia or nephrolithasis.

Timing

Haematuria at *beginning* of micturition: urethral.
Haematuria *throughout* micturition: bladder.
Haematuria at *end* of micturition: upper renal tract.

Colour of urine

Haematuria from a glomerular lesion may cause the urine to appear brown, green or tea-coloured.

Haematuria from a non-glomerular lesion may appear red-pink.

Past medical history

Certain medical conditions are associated with haematuria and these need to be excluded. They are:

sickle-cell disease
cystic kidney disease or renal tumours

systemic lupus erythematosus (SLE)

congenital heart disase (CHD) (e.g. immune complex glomeru-lonephritis associated with endocarditis)

malignancy, e.g. treatment with chemotherapy or radiotherapy

medications, e.g. aggressive use of frusemide (for instance in CHD or in the neonatal period) can cause hypercalciuria.

Family history

A detailed family history should be taken. Several conditions that cause haematuria are genetic in origin, e.g. Alport's syndrome (hearing loss and renal failure), polycystic kidney disease, sickle-cell disease.

Nephrolithiasis and IgA nephropathy also have familial association.

Social history

Non-accidental injury needs to be considered in the differential diagnosis if the cause of haematuria is thought to be trauma (see Chapter 26).

Examination

Examination should be full, as outlined in Chapters 2 and 3. Certain points deserve specific mention.

- **Basic observations**: a full set of observations should be taken. In particular, the presence of **increased blood pressure** should alert one to the possibility of a more severe underlying condition.
- **Head, ENT**: **oedema** frequently is observed first as swelling around the eyes. **Fundoscopy** may reveal signs of **hypertension**, if long-standing. **Erythema** or **exudate** of the pharynx may reveal streptococcal disease (although post-streptococcal glomeruloneph-ritis usually occurs at least 7 days after infection).
- **Chest, cardiovascular system**: Examine for evidence of **fluid overload**, such as **rales**, **gallop rhythm** or displaced **cardiac impulse.**

  Evidence of serositis such as **rubs** can help identify SLE or uraemia.
- **Abdomen**: a careful examination for **masses** is critical for the iden-tification of malignancy and polycystic kidney disease. **Ascites** sug-gests nephrosis. **Renal bruits** are audible in renal vascular disease.

Loin/flank tenderness often is seen in infection and **distention** from urethral obstruction.

- **Genitourinary system**: the genitalia should be examined for **trauma, discharge** and **meatal stenosis**.
- **Limbs**: examine for **oedema** or signs of **arthritis**.
- **Skin**: evaluate any **rashes** presenting with haematuria, particularly for signs of **skin infection, purpura/petechiae** or **malar rash**.

Investigations

Urinary dipstick tests

Despite the fact that they are very sensitive (and therefore not entirely reliable) urine dipsticks are the first investigation in any child presenting with haematuria. In addition to identifying possible blood in the urine the dipsticks are useful for indentifying **proteinuria**. In the absence of gross haematuria, proteinuria > 2+ by dipstick indicates a *glomerular* cause of haematuria. Haematuria without proteinuria of unknown cause in 50% will clear spontaneously.

Urine microscopy

In addition to confirming the presence of red blood cells, certain other information can be gained from urine microscopy. The presence of **red cell casts** indicates an intrarenal cause (either glomerular or tubular) and red cells may be **dysmorphic** due to distortion as they pass through the glomerular capillary wall. Glomerular casts indicate a glomerular cause. **Pyuria** and **bacteriuria** point to an infective cause (which should be confirmed by culture). Microscopy may also (rarely) identify the ova of *Schistosoma* if there has been recent travel to the tropics.

Other tests

Further investigation is dependent upon history, examination and urinalysis and microscopy. The management algorithm (Fig. 8.1) guides investigations.

- **Urine culture** – in almost all cases. This will confirm bacterial infection and lead to appropriate further investigations.

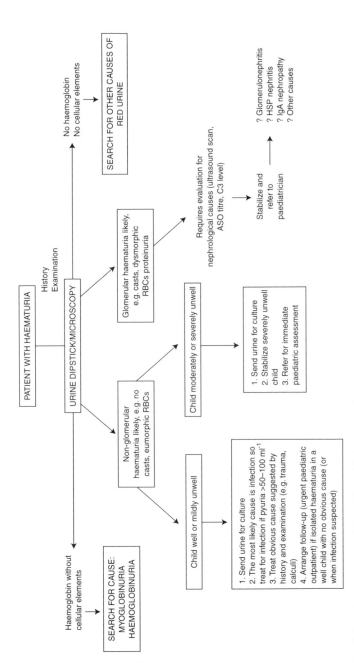

Fig. 8.1 *Management of the child with haematuria.*

ASO, antistreptolysin O; HSP, Henoch–Schönlein purpura; IgA, immunoglobulin A; RBC, red blood cells.

- **Full blood count**, **film** and **coagulation tests** – to exclude co-agulopathy and sickle-cell disease.
- **Radiology** – an abdominal ultrasound scan may identify a renal mass, evidence of obstruction or renal tract calculus. Calculi are occasionally seen on plain abdominal X-rays, but intravenous urography may be needed to confirm the site of obstruction.
- Further investigations for glomerulonephritis may include:
  - plasma urea and electrolytes, creatinine
  - calcium
  - phosphate
  - antistreptolysin O (ASO) and anti-DNA titres
  - complement screen
  - autoantibody screen

MANAGEMENT AND REFERRAL

Management is directed towards whether:

1. The patient is symptomatic or asymptomatic.
2. The presentation is acute, subacute or chronic.

The principles of management are outlined in the algorithm in Fig. 8.1.

> All causes of haematuria accompanied by oedema, oliguria, hypertension or significant proteinuria should be referred for immediate paediatric advice

OUTCOME AND PROGNOSIS

The outcome and prognosis are dependent on the diagnosis, but remember that most children will be well and the most common causes (e.g. infection) are usually dealt with easily.

OEDEMA

BACKGROUND INFORMATION

- Oedema is caused by excessive interstitial fluid and may be localized or generalized.
- Clinical assessment is directed towards determining whether transudation or exudation is likely and whether the problem is primarily renal or attributable to some other cause (e.g. hepatic or intestinal).
- Causes of oedema are outlined in Box 8.2.

Box 8.2 *Causes of oedema*

1. Decreased oncotic pressure, usually due to hypoproteinaemia (e.g. nephrotic syndrome, burns, protein-losing malabsorption states)

2. Increased capillary permeability (e.g. allergy, burns, trauma)

3. Increased capillary pressure (e.g. cardiac failure)

4. Lymphatic blockage (e.g. malignancy, post-surgical)

DIAGNOSTIC APPROACH

A practical approach to the assessment of oedema is to determine (by history, examination or investigation) the answers to the following questions:

- Is the swelling localized or generalized? If localized, this suggests an inflammatory cause, or occasionally immobility.
- If the swelling is more widespread, is there any proteinuria (and hypoproteinaemia)? If so, this suggests nephrotic syndrome.
- If there is *no* proteinuria but more widespread swelling, there may be several possible causes.
  1. Cardiac or lymphatic causes would not be associated with hypoproteinaemia.

2. Intestinal causes (malabsorption, protein-losing enteropathy, malnutrition), hepatic causes or sepsis may be associated with hypoproteinaemia.
3. Allergy.

History

Children are most likely to present with 'swelling'. Questions to be asked include:

- Is the swelling **localized** or **generalized**, and **where** and **when** did it start? Rapid onset of local oedema suggests allergy; immobility is often associated with oedema of the **lower limbs**. Generalized oedema is usually first noted on the **face**, often when the child **wakes in the morning**. Beware cases of 'allergy' with swollen eyes and face – consider nephrotic syndrome and check for proteinuria. Oedema of the lower parts of the body, including the **scrotum**, may only become apparent later in the day.
- Is the oedema **mild** or **severe**?
- Are there **associated symptoms**? **Skin rash** may occur as part of an allergic reaction (**urticaria**), particularly if associated with **itch**. **Facial oedema** with **stridor** may suggest impending respiratory compromise. **Fever** may indicate infection, particularly if associated with **redness**.

Examination

- **Basic observations** should be recorded: **fever** should be confirmed; **tachycardia** may occur in response to infection, anaphylaxis or in cases of significant volume depletion as might occur in hypoproteinaemic oedema; **hypertension** is an adverse prognostic factor in cases of oedema due to nephrotic syndrome, may indicate nephritis in Henoch–Schönlein purpura, or may simply be a response to stress.
- General observations should include an assessment of whether the child looks **toxic** (peritonitis is a complication of nephrotic syndrome) or **malnourished** (malabsorption), although oedema is rarely the presenting feature of malabsorption states. **Rashes**

should be sought: **petechiae** on the **extensor surfaces** point to Henoch–Schönlein purpura, **urticaria** indicates allergy.

- Oedema should be assessed to see if it is **pitting** or **non-pitting**, the latter possibly indicating a chronic problem of lymphatics or associated with denervation. Lymphatic pathology is usually hereditary and rare in childhood, as too is oedema due to **congestive cardiac failure**. The **areas affected** must be noted for the reasons already outlined.
- Chronic liver disease may manifest with **veins** on the **anterior abdominal wall** or **spider naevi** and examination of the abdomen should include assessment of **liver size**. **Splenomegaly** may indicate portal hypertension. **Ascites** should be sought.
- Cardiovascular disease should be considered by checking for the presence of pleural or pericardial **effusions**.
- Localized limb swelling should raise suspicion of trauma as the cause (see Chapters 15 and 16).

Investigations

The most important investigation in the A&E department is **urinalysis.**

- Heavy proteinuria immediately points to a diagnosis of nephrotic syndrome.
- Moderate proteinuria with heavy haematuria suggests glomerulonephritis.
- Absent or minimal proteinuria suggests a non-renal cause.

Other investigations would be directed by the clinical findings and paediatric or senior A&E staff, but might well include a **full blood count** (particularly if infection is implicated), **urea and electrolytes**, **liver function tests** (to confirm hypoproteinaemia) and other blood tests when nephrotic syndrome is suspected (e.g. **ASO titre, antinuclear antibodies**). **Urine culture** should be carried out to exclude infection.

MANAGEMENT AND REFERRAL

- Local oedema from allergic responses can be treated with **anti-histamines** (e.g. chlorpheniramine syrup) or, if an anaphylactic response, in the manner described on p. 234.
- Oedema from other obvious causes (e.g. burns or trauma) should be treated according to guidelines outlined in the appropriate chapter.
- Oedema of all other types should be **referred** for paediatric assessment.

OUTCOME AND PROGNOSIS

The outcome and prognosis depend upon the precise diagnosis. However, even in cases of nephrotic syndrome, the prognosis can be good.

If the child is under 5 years old, blood pressure and levels of urea, electrolytes and creatinine are normal, and there is no haematuria, the underlying condition is likely to be minimal change nephritis, and empiric treatment with steroids (under the guidance of a paediatric nephrologist) will often be very successful. Even if relapse occurs, death from complications is rare. Nephrotic syndrome from other causes may cause renal failure.

9 CHILDREN PRESENTING WITH TOXIC INGESTION

BACKGROUND INFORMATION

Suspected poisoning in children is a common problem in A&E departments. It presents as:

- **Accidental ingestion** – inquisitive and inadequately supervised toddlers.
- **Deliberate self-harm** – distressed or disturbed children, generally older than 10 years.
- **Deliberate poisoning** – Munchausen syndrome by proxy (rare), dependent children (attention seeking parents).

General principles of care involve:

1. The re-establishment of vital functions and supportive measures.
2. Identification of the poison.
3. Attempted elimination of the poison:
        adsorption of toxin in bowel
        irrigation of the stomach
        specific antidotes
        increased rate of excretion

RESUSCITATION

Following accidental ingestion the child is likely to be completely well. However, severe illness, unconsciousness, fitting or other complications may follow ingestion of a serious toxin such as a tricyclic antidepressant. In such cases, call for help and assess and support:
        airway
        breathing
        circulation

Then check:

> **responsiveness** (AVPU)
> **blood glucose level**

For the management of fits see Chapter 22 but use no more medication than is necessary as this may aggravate the toxic state.

DIAGNOSTIC APPROACH

History

Identify:

> **what has been taken**
> **how much has been taken**
> **at what time this occurred**
> **how did it occur** (looking at accident prevention)

If the parent telephones before bringing the child, request that the packet or bottle (or sample of plant material, e.g. berries) is brought with them. Although experience shows that *accidental* ingestion of paracetamol is not normally toxic, treat according to the worse scenario if there is uncertainty about timing or quantity.

Remember that in deliberate self-harm, you are not always told the truth. Find out if previous attempts have occurred. What has precipitated this episode? Is there a real danger of suicide?

If a toxin is identified, obtain advice from a poisons information centre or database. There are eight recognized poisons information centres in the British Isles which can provide telephone advice day and night. The numbers are listed in the *British National Formulary* section on the emergency treatment of poisoning.

> **IT IS ALWAYS ADVISABLE TO CHECK WITH A POISONS INFORMATION CENTRE FOR UP-TO-DATE ADVICE**

Examination

In the stable child who does not require resuscitation, perform a rapid **top to toe examination**.

Investigations

Investigations other than those needed for intensive management of a seriously ill child (see Chapter 22) will be highlighted in advice from a poisons unit. **Blood** (up to 10 ml in a plain tube) and **urine** for toxicology screening should be obtained in any child in whom deliberate or serious accidental poisoning is suspected.

The most frequent investigation performed is assessment of the paracetamol level at 4 h post ingestion which helps to determine the need for further treatment with *N*-acetylcysteine (see below).

Diagnosis

The diagnosis is usually self-evident, but consider poisoning as a diagnosis in any child whose cause of unconsciousness is unknown.

MANAGEMENT AND REFERRAL

It is important to ensure that treatment is needed for the substance ingested – this is often not the case in children.

Elimination of poison

- **Emesis** using ipecacuanha ('ipecac') syrup may be useful in the primary care setting if it is known that a child has ingested sufficient material within the preceding 2–3 h to produce a toxic effect and that access to further treatment will take another couple of hours. Ipecac takes 20 min to induce vomiting. IT IS STRONGLY CONTRAINDICATED if the child is obtunded or becoming less responsive, and also if a petroleum distillate has been ingested as there is then a risk of aspiration pneumonitis.
- **Adsorption** of the toxin with oral charcoal (effective against a multitude of chemicals) has now superseded emesis. If charcoal is necessary but the child will not drink it, it can be administered through a nasogastric tube (dose of charcoal, 1 mg kg^{-1}). Exceptionally, induction of anaesthesia may be justified, but this decison can only be taken by an experienced paediatrician.

- **Gastric lavage** can be performed if ingestion has occurred within the preceding 4 to 6 h and the child is known to have taken a potentially serious amount of toxin. Though it is of most benefit if performed within 1–2 h of ingestion, drugs that are slow to leave the stomach (e.g. aspirin or anticholinergics such as tricyclic antidepressants) may be effectively removed by lavage within 12 h. If the nature of the poison is unknown, the gastric fluid can be sent for toxicological analysis. If the child is already obtunded, paediatric advice must be sought and lavage not attempted before an anaesthetist has assessed the airway, and secured it if necessary with a tracheal tube. Charcoal should usually be administered down the gastric lavage tube just before it is removed.

Specific poisons

The management of some specific common or serious poisonings is shown below.

Paracetamol

The liver damage (hepatocellular necrosis) induced by serious paracetamol overdose is maximal on the third to fourth day after ingestion. Rarely renal tubular necrosis also occurs. Symptoms of overdose are miminal, often allowing the patient to be falsely reassured. In normal children, no danger is seen with doses of less than 150 mg kg^{-1}.

The plasma **paracetamol concentration** is measured at 4 h (or longer) to gauge the need for treatment with *N*-acetylcysteine (NAC) and specialist referral. Paracetamol toxicity graphs are freely available in A&E departments, the *British National Formulary* or the packets of NAC. Paracetamol toxicity is more likely if **malnutrition** or **enzyme-inducing agents** (carbamazepine, phenytoin, phenobarbitone, rifampicin) are involved.

Tricyclic antidepressants

Tricyclic antidepressants are a common source of toxic ingestion in childhood, the main manifestations being coma, tachycardia and arrhythmias, hypotension, hypothermia, hyperreflexia with extensor plantar responses, and respiratory failure.

Treatment is directed towards correction of any metabolic acidosis, hypoxia, hypothermia, etc. Diazepam may be helpful in terminating convulsions. Delirium and hallucinations may occur during the recovery phase. Cardiotoxicity is reduced by increasing blood pH. Specialist referral is mandatory.

Iron poisoning

Poisoning with iron is surprisingly common in toddlers – largely because they take their mother's antenatal iron/folate preparations. Iron in toxic amounts causes manifestations of nausea, vomiting, abdominal pain and diarrhoea. Haematemesis, rectal bleeding, hypotension, coma and hepatocellular necrosis may follow.

Treatment consists of specialist referral prior to gastric lavage and administration of the antidote, desferrioxamine. The serum iron level is a good indicator of toxicity but when this is expected to be high, treatment should start before the result is available.

> ANY CHILD WHOSE INGESTION OR EXPOSURE IS POTENTIALLY TOXIC MUST BE REFERRED FOR SPECIALIST PAEDIATRIC CARE

Deliberate poisoning

Older children who have deliberately taken a substance thought to be harmful should always be referred for a psychiatric evaluation. The adolescent who presents repeatedly with self-harm is not easily assessed or treated in a busy A&E department. Do remember that there is often a significant, perhaps undisclosed, reason for this person's unhappiness, and make every attempt to involve others who could be helpful (sympathetic nursing staff, social worker, community paediatrician, schoolteacher, etc.).

Deliberate poisoning by carers is often very hard to diagnose because the efforts made to deceive all involved are sometimes taken to the extreme. Physical damage may result from repeated life-threatening episodes.

OUTCOME AND PROGNOSIS

More than 50% of children exposed to a potential poison are completely unaffected as either the substance or the amount is harmless. For the remainder, the prognosis depends on the substance, the dose involved, time before treatment, the effectiveness of elimination techniques and the child's general health.

In all instances, prevention of such episodes must at some stage be discussed with the parents and the health visitor needs to be informed.

10 CHILDREN WITH NEUROLOGICAL SYMPTOMS

Acute neurological presentations other than convulsions, are rare in childhood. Convulsions are also described in Chapters 5 and 22. This chapter discusses the management of short and completed convulsions, as well as faints and 'funny turns' which are not usually of cardiac origin in children (unlike adults). However, cardiac causes need occasionally to be considered.

Any child with more unusual neurological presentations should be referred for paediatric assessment.

FITS, FAINTS AND FUNNY TURNS

BACKGROUND INFORMATION

Fits in childhood are common. As many as 1 in 100 children will have a nonfebrile seizure at some stage. However, some abnormal episodes are wrongly labelled as epilepsy (e.g. reflex anoxic seizures, breath-holding attacks, simple faints). A true fit will normally interrupt the behaviour or play that was previously being exhibited.

DIAGNOSTIC APPROACH

History

When a child presents following an episode that may have been a fit, an accurate history from an eye-witness is of utmost importance. For example:

- What was the child **doing beforehand**?

- What was the exact **sequence of events** within the episode?
- What was its **duration**?
- How **sudden was the onset** and how **rapid the recovery**?
- Was the child **sleepy** after the event?
- Does the child have any **recollection** of the event?

Check for:

- **Family history** of seizures.
- **Predisposing factors** (e.g. fever in the age range 6 months to 6 years, see p. 27)
- Underlying **developmental abnormality**.
- History of **neonatal problems, other illness** or **fits**.
- **Other symptoms** (e.g. palpitations).

Examination

A full examination of the child is necessary, paying special attention to the level of consciousness and the neurological examination. A temporal assessment of conscious level will allow recovery to be evaluated.

Investigations

If a child has fully recovered and this is an isolated incident, no investigation is necessary other than routine nursing observations including the blood pressure.

If the history suggests a fainting episode, check for any hypotension (blood pressure lying and standing).

If the history suggests a primary cardiac event (e.g. arrhythmia), a baseline ECG will be essential.

If there are recurring episodes, the electrolytes, calcium and magnesium levels should be checked.

If the child is on anticonvulsant medicine such as carbamazepine, phenytoin or phenobarbitone, drug levels may be useful to the GP. If they are measured, the results must be communicated to the child's GP or paediatrician.

MANAGEMENT AND REFERRAL

If the child recovers fully after a period of observation, there is no need for immediate action but it may be advisable to discuss with paediatric staff.

For a first seizure or when there is any doubt about the cause of the 'funny turn', outpatient referral to a paediatrician can be recommended (usually through the GP). The referral needs to contain a record of the A&E history (as above).

Any child who has a prolonged seizure (over 20 min), who does not fully recover, or in whom there are persistent neurological signs, needs to be referred to senior staff or a paediatrician for assessment and admission.

OUTCOME AND PROGNOSIS

Outcome depends on the underlying diagnosis.

11 CHILDREN PRESENTING WITH A RASH

BACKGROUND INFORMATION

Skin rashes are a common cause for concern amongst parents.

A rash may be due to an intrinsic skin disease (e.g. psoriasis, eczema); it may be secondary to a systemic illness (e.g. Henoch–Schönlein purpura, Kawasaki's disease); or it may be caused by an external insult to a localized area of skin, such as infection (e.g. impetigo), infestation (e.g. scabies) or burns.

Rashes may be transient and insignificant, or of great importance as indicators of severe underlying disease.

DIAGNOSTIC APPROACH

History

Use initial questions to establish the **child's general condition** (see Chapters 2 and 3).

Record:

> **onset** of rash
>
> **symptoms** of rash – e.g. itchy, blistering, evanescent (come and go in minutes)
>
> **progress** – e.g. worsening, improving?
>
> nature of any **previous episodes**?
>
> personal or family history of **atopy**?
>
> exposure to **irritants/allergens**
>
> **contact with infection**, e.g. chickenpox
>
> **medication**
>
> **any treatment tried**
>
> any features of **systemic disease**

Examination

Note the child's general condition. Look for any **underlying illness**. Is there a **fever**? Check the **pulse** and **respiratory rate**.

Look specifically for **associated problems**, e.g. lymphadenopathy in Kawasaki's disease, infection in eczema, hepatosplenomegaly, pallor, and bruising in acute leukaemia.

Note the following points about the rash:

- **Site** and **distribution** of rash.
- **Description**:
    is the affected skin raised (papular), flat (macular), scaly and thickened (ichthyotic, lichenified), blistered (producing vesicles or bullae)?
    what is its colour?
    are the lesions confluent, discrete, evanescent, migratory (moving over a period of days)?

Investigations

Investigations for specific conditions are summarized in Table 11.1.

MANAGEMENT AND REFERRAL

See Table 11.1.

OUTCOME AND PROGNOSIS

Outcome and prognosis depend on the condition diagnosed.

Table 11.1 *Diagnosis and treatment of skin rashes*

Description	Distribution or other features	Possible diagnosis	Investigations	Treatment	Review
Vesicular	Dermatome	Shingles	Electron microscopy of fresh blister fluid Swab for viral culture (VZV)?	Acyclovir (topical/oral) **Beware immuno-compromised – must refer for advice**	Not required
Discrete vesicles (on a base of erythema)	Axial greater than acral	Chickenpox	As above (if any)	Rarely required **Beware immuno-compromised- must refer for advice**	Not required Secondary bacterial infection can occur; treat with oral antibiotic e.g. co-amoxiclav
Discrete vesicles	Palms, soles superficial oral ulceration/blisters	Hand, foot and mouth disease (coxsackie-virus)	As above (if any)	Topical anti-inflammatory for sore mouth (e.g. benzydamine oral spray)	Only if concerns about reduced fluid intake – generally only transient
Red, sore mouth	Superficial ulceration of oral mucosa including tongue	Herpes stomatitis (type 1)	Swab for viral culture Saliva for electron microscopy	Ensure hydration Oral acyclovir may hasten recovery	Only if concerns about reduced fluid intake – generally only transient

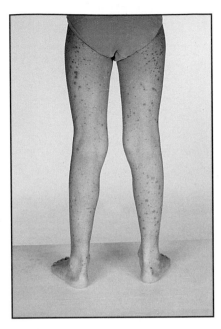

Plate 1. Classic distribution and rash as seen in Henoch-Schönlein purpura.

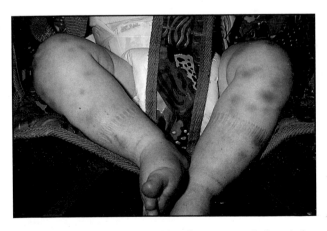

Plate 2. Multiple bruising on shins in a non-ambulant infant. Idiopathic thrombocytopenia purpura was the diagnosis but consider non-accidental injury.

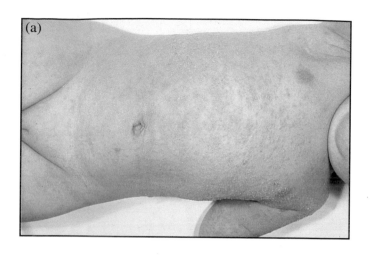

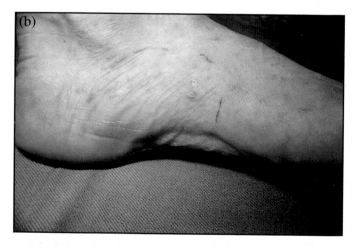

Plate 3. (a) Scabetic rash in infants. (b) Scabetic burrow on instep of foot in an older child.

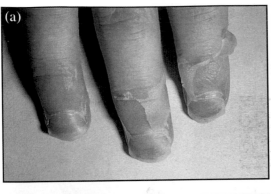

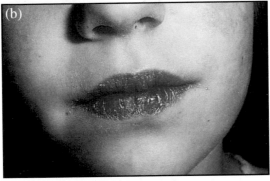

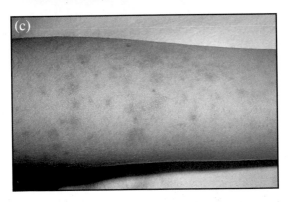

Plate 4. Kawasaki's disease (mucocutaneous lymph node syndrome). (a) Fingers peeling. (b) Sore dry lips. (c) Widespread macular rash.

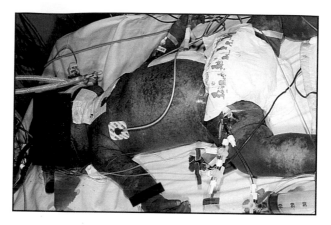

Plate 5. Purpuric rash in severe meningococcal septicaemia. Petechiae, purpurae or this widespread purpuric rash can be seen or the atypical evanescent macular rash that may fade.

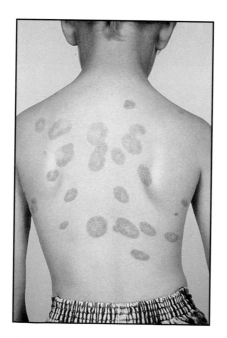

Plate 6. Classic psoriatic rash.

Table 11.1 *Continued*

Description	Distribution or other features	Possible diagnosis	Investigations	Treatment	Review
Maculopapular (coarse)	Generalized rash, Koplik's spots on buccal mucosa, pink conjunctivae, otitis media	Measles	Nil	Nil. Generalized supportive treatment may be required in unwell children	Rarely required. Measles is seen extremely rarely in the UK thanks to effective vaccine
Maculopapular (fine)	Trunk more than limbs	Non-specific viral rash (child otherwise well)	Nil	Nil	Nil
Widespread macular rash, red palms	Conjunctival inflammation, red, sore, cracked lips, persistent high fever, generalized lymphadenopathy	Kawasaki's disease (mucocutaneous lymph node syndrome) skin of fingers peels later	Refer for specialist opinion (thrombocytosis develops after 2 weeks)	Specialist paediatric management (intravenous immunoglobulin). Coronary artery aneurysms occur rarely (by 4 weeks)	Cardiac ultrasound scan at 4 weeks – repeat after further 4 weeks
Generalized red skin	Conjuctivae and oral mucosa **spared**. Sometimes characteristic superficial cracking around nasolabial region/upper lip	Staphylococcal 'scalded skin' syndrome. Skin subsequently shows superficial peeling	If child is unwell refer for advice, full blood count, CRP, blood cultures. Look for source of staphylococcal infection	Fluxoxacillin (rarely modifies this toxin-induced condition). iv fluids may be required	Refer

Table 11.1 *Diagnosis and treatment of skin rashes* (continued)

Description	Distribution or other features	Possible diagnosis	Investigations	Treatment	Review
Red skin, red eyes, sore mouth	Generalized erythema, unwell	Stevens–Johnson syndrome (severe erythema multiforme)	Refer for supportive treatment	Give oral/iv fluids, maintain body temperature, ensure adequate energy intake, systemic steroids may be used but evidence of benefit is equivocal	Refer for specialist management
Target lesions	Patchy or generalized – discrete lesions may coalesce	Erythema multiforme	Avoidance of any recognized trigger	Nil	Nil Warn parents to seek help if condition worsens (see Stevens–Johnson syndrome above)

Signs	Condition	Distribution	Investigations	Treatment	Notes
Erythema, ulcerated/weeping, evidence of dry skin elsewhere	Eczema (atopic dermatitis)	Classically in flexures of limbs, around root of ears, hands look for cradle cap – erythema also more generalized in infants	Nil Swab for MC&S if appears infected	Emollient creams (e.g. E45, Unguentum Merck, Diprobase) Avoidance of saponifying agents (use aqueous cream, Oilatum Emollient, Balneum for bath) Topical steroid – minimum strength to control activity	Often managed by GP refer to dermatologist if regular use of strong topical steroids required.
Hyperkeratotic papules	Psoriasis	Classically extensor aspect of limbs, scalp Guttate pattern more widespread (Koebner's phenomenon)	Nil	Specific dermatological treatment (topical tar preparations, PUVA)	Can be difficult to recognize in infancy Can present as erythroderma
Bluish erythematous nodules	Erythema nodosum	Shins	(Can advise GP to) check for evidence of recent streptococcal disease and viral serology	Nil	Refer if history of chronic underlying disease, e.g. inflammatory bowel disease, tuberculosis

Table 11.1 *Diagnosis and treatment of skin rashes* (continued)

Description	Distribution or other features	Possible diagnosis	Investigations	Treatment	Review
Purple blotches, non-blanching	Backs of legs, buttocks, shins, forearms	Henoch–Schönlein purpura	Urinalysis (blood and protein) Full blood count if diagnosis unsure (cf ITP below)	Refer and observe if complications of 1. Intussussception 2. Renal involvement (significant urinary residue, hypertension)	Rash, synovial swelling, epididymitis tend to settle spontaneously If small amounts of pro-teinuria and haematuria and BP normal, reanalyse after 1 week and refer for advice if necessary
Non-blanching purpura, petechiae, poor limb perfusion	Generalized rash, child **unwell**, fever, tachycardia	Meningococcal septicaemia	CALL FOR HELP (blood cultures, full blood count, CRP, U&E, bicarbonate, calcium, clotting screen, group and save serum, EDTA sample for PCR)	Oxygen, colloid, cefotaxime Refer	Managed as in-patient

Multiple bruises with or without petechiae	Generalized	Idiopathic thrombocytopenic purpura	Full blood count Spontaneous bruising occurs with platelet count $< 20 \times 10^9 \, l^{-1}$	Refer for advice Differential diagnosis includes NAI	Spontaneous resolution most common
Petechiae	Around eyelids, facial	Induced by coughing or vomiting	Nil	Nil	Nil
Petechiae	In linear pattern	Induced by scratching	Nil	Nil	Nil
Papular, itchy red rash associated with white (histaminic) papules	Trunk or limbs	Urticaria	Nil	Oral +/– topical antihistamines to reduce itching	Nil
Pruritic excoriated lesions	Finger webs, volar aspect of forearm May be widespread in babies	Scabies	Possible to winkle out mite from burrow	Acaricides (treatment for babies may differ from adults – consult current local guidelines)	Itch will not resolve for several days Itch helped by calamine lotion
Red, scaly, discrete, occasionally bullous	Face, limbs, groin	Impetigo	Skin swab for MC&S (staphylococcal)	Oral antibiotics (fluxoxacillin or co-amoxiclav) If widespread Topical application (sodium fusidate ointment)	Nil

Table 11.1 *Diagnosis and treatment of skin rashes* (continued)

Description	Distribution or other features	Possible diagnosis	Investigations	Treatment	Review
Warm, erythematous, swollen epidermis and dermis	Anywhere	Cellulitis	Full blood count, blood cultures if unwell	Oral or parenteral antibiotics (penicillin, co-amoxiclav) Orbital cellulitis: use co-amoxiclav (anaerobic and *Haemophilus* cover)	Refer any unwell child Refer orbital cellulitis
Superficial, enlarging scaly ring	Trunk or limbs	Ringworm	Skin scrapings for fungal recognition if not responding to treatment	Topical antifungal agent, e.g. clotrimazole	Nil

BP, blood pressure; CRP, C-reactive protein; GP, general practitioner; ITP, idiopathic thrombocytopenic purpura; IV, intravenous; MC&S, microscopy, culture and sensitivities; NAI, non-accidental injury; PCR, polymerase chain reaction; PUVA, psoralens with ultraviolet A; VZV, varicella-zoster virus

12 CHILDREN WITH EAR, NOSE AND THROAT SYMPTOMS

Diseases of the ear, nose, throat (ENT) and mouth are considered together, as symptoms or signs at one of these sites is often due to disease of another. Common symptoms that present to the A&E department include the following:

sore throat
aural discharge
hearing loss
foreign body (nose/ear)
epistaxis
nasal discharge
earache

Each of these symptoms is considered in this chapter. Stridor is considered in Chapter 6. Foreign bodies are considered in Chapter 28.

Other symptoms, such as cough, fever and headache may also be a feature of ENT conditions. At all times, therefore, the possibility of a *systemic* disorder should be considered, and a proper clinical history and examination will extend well beyond the ears, nose and throat (see Chapters 2 and 3).

SORE THROAT

BACKGROUND INFORMATION

- Sore throat is very common in childhood. Acute infection of the upper respiratory tract affects the average child approximately four times per year.
- A sore throat is a result of inflammation of the pharyngeal mucosa, occasionally caused by trauma but usually due to infective agents.

- The main difficulty lies in differentiating between viral and bacterial infections of the upper respiratory tract. The differential diagnosis includes pharyngitis, acute tonsillitis, quinsy and infectious mononucleosis.
- The majority of sore throats (60%) are caused by viral infections including the common cold, adenoviruses, influenza/parainfluenza viruses, coxsackieviruses and echoviruses. Of the remainder, the majority are caused by group A beta-haemolytic streptococci, although infection with this micro-organism is uncommon in children less than 3 years old.

DIAGNOSTIC APPROACH

Unfortunately there is no absolutely reliable clinical way of determining whether a child is suffering from a viral or bacterial infection. The following features may aid the diagnosis. However, even in viral infection, secondary bacterial infection can occur.

History

Sore throat is often described but its presence in the younger child may need to be inferred from the presence of **fever**, **refusal of food** or **drooling**.

Age

- Viral infections occur at any age, whereas acute bacterial tonsillitis is commonest at approximately 4–6 years of age.
- Acute tonsillitis then lessens in frequency and severity over a period of 2–3 years and it becomes increasingly uncommon after 10 years of age.
- Infectious mononucleosis (glandular fever), although it can occur at any age, is more common in adolescence.

Duration of symptoms

- Although an imprecise guide, the onset of sore throat in acute tonsillitis is frequently more sudden, developing over a period of hours to a day, compared with the more gradual onset of the typically minor sore throat in acute viral pharyngitis.

- In glandular fever, malaise and lethargy may have accompanied a sore throat of varying severity over a period of several days.

Associated symptoms

- **Sneezing**, **runny nose** (coryza) and **runny eyes** (due to oedema of the nasolacrimal duct) are all symptoms that suggest a generalized viral upper respiratory tract infection.

- **Pain radiating to the ears**, in the absence of acute otitis media, occurs most commonly in acute bacterial tonsillitis rather than in viral upper respiratory tract infections, although it may be a feature of both.

- **Fever** is a common feature of all causes of sore throat in childhood. The degree of fever cannot reliably be used to determine whether the infection is viral or bacterial. However, a high fever (greater than 38.5°C) is generally associated with a greater degree of systemic upset and may increase the tendency to prescribe antibiotics.

- **Painful neck** is a common feature of all respiratory tract infections and is related to cervical lymphadenopathy. It is particularly marked in acute bacterial tonsillitis and infectious mononucleosis, and occasionally the associated stiff neck is interpreted as 'meningism'.

- **Rashes** increase the likelihood of an underlying *viral* illness. Sore throat can be a feature of measles infection but measles-like rashes are now more common in (non-specific) viral illnesses or infectious mononucleosis, particularly if amoxycillin or ampicillin has been prescribed. Occasionally a rash will appear uniformly red and be accompanied by a **sore tongue** with enlarged papillae. This raises the possibility of scarlet fever (caused by erythrogenic beta-haemolytic streptococcus) and occasionally pathognomonic **striae** may be seen on the flexor aspect of the elbows.

- **Trismus** (spasm of the masseter muscle) raises the possibility of quinsy.

- **Cough** may be evidence of lower respiratory tract involvement.

- **Abdominal pain** can be a feature of acute tonsillitis or infectious mononucleosis in the older child, but occasionally indicates a lower respiratory infection.

Examination

Basic observations should be recorded: **pulse** and **temperature** are both typically raised. An increased **respiratory rate** may indicate lower respiratory tract involvement or simply reflect fever in the younger child.

ENT examination

There is no easy way to differentiate a viral from a bacterial cause of sore throat by examination.

Pharynx, tonsils
- **Exudate** should be noted but the presence of pus can be a feature of both viral and bacterial pharyngitis and tonsillitis.
- In acute pharyngitis the throat often looks **hyperaemic**, whereas in acute tonsillitis hyperaemia is **centred around the tonsils**.
- **Unilateral tonsillar enlargement**, particularly if associated with trismus, may indicate quinsy.

Palate, cheeks
- A **petechial rash** on the palate can be a feature of streptococcal infection and glandular fever.
- **Ulcers on the fauces** may indicate coxsackie virus infection.
- **Koplik's spots** are discrete white nodules with a surrounding area of erythema on the mucosa of the inside of the cheek and palate, and indicate measles when accompanied by acute pharyngitis, particularly if there is also a cough.

Nose
A **runny nose** should be noted as this is generally taken to be an indicator of viral infection.

Neck
Cervical lymph nodes are generally enlarged and tender in all causes of sore throat, but particularly in glandular fever.

Note: there is no 'normal size' for tonsils and apparent enlargement is not an indication of past or even current infection. Hypertrophy of lymph gland tissue (tonsils, adenoids, cervical lymph nodes) is a normal part of the development of immunocompetence in childhood and is not pathological.

Systemic examination

Skin
The **distribution** and **description of any rash** should be recorded (see Chapter 11) and skin should be examined (along with fontanelle and eyes) for dehydration (see Chapter 2).

Chest
Examination of the lower respiratory tract should be carried out to exclude the **signs of lower respiratory tract infection** (see Chapter 6).

Abdomen
Generalized **abdominal tenderness** can be a feature of upper respiratory tract infections in general, but particularly acute tonsillitis. The liver and spleen may be tender and occasionally **enlarged** in glandular fever.

Investigations

Investigations are generally *unnecessary* in most cases of sore throat. The following may be helpful:

- **Full blood count**: a marked lymphocytosis with atypical lymphocytes may indicate glandular fever.
- **Throat swab**: although it is unlikely to alter management, a swab of the patient's throat can allow the doctor to assess whether the clinical diagnosis is correct, and is usually considered advisable prior to commencing antibiotics (where these are indicated).
- **Monospot/Paul–Bunnell test** may be positive, indicating glandular fever.

- **Viral antibody studies** may be necessary in chronic cases of sore throat.
- **Chest X-ray** may be helpful, particularly in the younger child, if a lower respiratory tract infection needs to be excluded.

MANAGEMENT AND REFERRAL

- Most sore throats are managed with supportive treatment; adequate fluid intake (including an allowance for fever) and paracetamol or ibuprofen should be prescribed for fever and discomfort.
- In suspected viral infection, antibiotics have no part to play unless secondary bacterial infection causes complications (e.g. acute otitis media) and even then many practitioners doubt their role. Certainly antibiotics have no role in preventing such complications.
- In acute tonsillitis antibiotics are of value if there is significant *systemic* upset and should be considered if the child looks unwell despite antipyretic therapy, particularly if there is high fever (greater than 38.5°C). In these instances, oral penicillin V is the drug of choice and should be prescribed for 10 days, although most patients will be symptomatically better in 2–3 days. Failure to show improvement within 48 h of commencing penicillin indicates that the infection is viral or that the possibility of quinsy should be considered. Ampicillin and amoxycillin may be used for acute tonsillitis but they can worsen the rash associated with glandular fever. For a patient who is sensitive to penicillin, erythromycin is the alternative. Unless the child worsens or shows only very slow improvement, there is no indication for follow-up after the treatment of tonsillitis.
- Quinsy is an abscess of one of the tonsils and needle aspiration or surgical drainage is occasionally required. However, antibiotic treatment may be appropriate in the early stages. Large doses of oral antibiotics should be prescribed as a chronic septic mass can result from inadequate dosage. Parenteral antibiotics are often needed as patients often refuse oral medication. The child should be referred for assessment by ENT surgeons.
- Referral to a paediatrician for admission of a child with sore throat is rarely necessary and is reserved for cases of doubtful diagnosis, severe systemic upset or dehydration.

OUTCOME AND PROGNOSIS

The majority of sore throats settle irrespective of treatment. Complications following streptococcal infection are now rare in the UK as rheumatic fever is very uncommon, but occasional cases of post-streptococcal glomerulonephritis are seen. The malaise of glandular fever can last for several months but usually resolves spontaneously.

EAR PAIN

BACKGROUND INFORMATION

- Ear pain is a very common symptom in childhood; by far the most common cause is acute otitis media. This is a bacterial infection of the middle ear and mastoid air system, occurring primarily in infants and young children, presenting with malaise, pyrexia and occasionally discharge.
- Spontaneous resolution often occurs with rupture and drainage through the tympanic membrane.
- *Rarely* drainage from mastoid air cells becomes blocked, causing an abscess within the mastoid, suspected clinically from **tenderness** and **swelling** over the mastoid area.
  Complications rarely include meningitis and brain abscess.
- *Causes*: viral URTI or bacterial infection (streptococci 20%, staphylococci 5%, pneumococci 30% and *Haemophilus influenzae* 5%). Commoner in children under 8 years old owing to relatively poor eustachian tube function: peak age 6–36 months (acute otitis media occurring in two-thirds by age of 3 years).
- Some children suffer recurrent otitis media with chronic middle ear effusion. Eustachian tube oedema is caused by the URTI. The child sleeps, mouth-breathes and does not swallow. Air is absorbed from the middle ear and a pressure differential develops across the tympanic membrane, causing otalgia. Passive smoking increases the risk, as does recurrent URTI and adenoidal hypertrophy. This can cause intermittent (but sometimes profound) hearing loss.

- It can be difficult to elucidate the cause of a painful ear, which can originate in the ear or temporomandibular joint, or be referred from elsewhere in the head and neck (Box 12.1).

Box 12.1 *Differential diagnosis of pain in the ear*

TYMPANIC MEMBRANE

otitis media

otitis media with effusion (glue ear)

bullous myringitis (related to *Mycoplasma* infection)

perforation

EXTERNAL EAR CANAL

foreign body

otitis externa

trauma

herpes simplex infection

herpes zoster infection

PINNA

sunburn

bites, boils, etc.

injury (including ear piercing)

REFERRED PAIN

tonsillitis

mumps/parotitis

lower teeth – teething, caries, developing molar teeth

cervical spine injury

ACUTE MASTOIDITIS

DIAGNOSTIC APPROACH

History

- The typical history is of a child, usually under 5 years old, waking in the middle of the night **screaming and crying** with **earache**.
- There is often preceding **cold or cough**, and the commonest diagnostic problem is distinguishing acute otitis media from glue ear, negative middle ear pressure and other upper respiratory tract or teeth causes.
- A history of **trauma** is usually obvious, as is a complaint of **discharge** (see below).
- Patients may occasionally present with **facial** or **neck swelling** (associated with ear pain), which may point to a diagnosis of viral parotitis.

Examination

A full examination should be carried out as outlined in Chapters 2 and 3, in particular looking for **rashes**, **swellings** and evidence of **trauma**.

Otoscopy

The technique for otoscopy is as follows:

1. Demonstrate the procedure to the small child on a parent, teddy-bear or doll.
2. Have the patient seated on the carer's lap, cuddled with one arm behind the carer's back.
3. Invite the carer to hold the child's head against the carer's chest, allowing visualization of each ear in turn.
4. The best view of the tympanic membrane (TM) is obtained in an infant by pulling the ear lobe downwards, and in a child by pulling the pinna up and back.

Common findings are summarized in Table 12.1

Table 12.1 *Common otoscopic findings*

Appearance	Diagnosis
Grey drum, cone of light reflex	Normal
Pink around rim of TM	Crying
Uniformly red and bulging	Acute otis media
Dark coloration or black	Blood behind TM or impending perforation
Black hole	Perforation
Dull grey, bulging, may show bubbles or fluid level (may be non-mobile on insufflation)	Secretory otis media
Red or discharging outer ear canal	Otitis externa
Dull grey, retracted	Blocked eustachian tube
Bullae on TM	Mycoplasma pneumoniae infection

Clinical diagnosis

In most cases simple diagnostic questions can be used.

1. Is the tympanic membrane bulging and red? If YES the child should be treated as having *acute otitis media*.
2. If not bulging and red, is the TM retracted? If YES, consider the possibility of *negative middle pressure and early otitis media with effusion*.
3. If the TM is neither retracted nor red and bulging (and there is no evidence of discharge) an *otological cause for the ear pain is unlikely*, so examine pharynx and teeth particularly.
4. If there is evidence of discharge, see next section (p. 130).

Investigations

Other investigations are rarely needed, but in addition to the guidelines outlined in Chapters 2 and 3 an **ear swab** for **microscopy**, **culture** and **sensitivity** may be useful if otitis externa is suspected, and a **skull X-ray** when there is a history of trauma or blood behind the tympanic membrane (although neuroimaging with **CT scan** has superseded this investigation).

MANAGEMENT AND REFERRAL

- The distinction between causes is not easy or relevant within the first 24 h, when analgesia is the priority. In most cases the pain will resolve, but if it persists an accurate diagnosis becomes more important.
- Specific details of management of otitis media and otitis media (with effusion) are given below.
- The management of otitis externa is covered on p. 132 and blood behind the TM secondary to trauma is covered in Chapter 23.
- If no obvious cause is found and the condition persists over 24 h, referral to a paediatrician or ENT specialist is appropriate.

Notes on other causes can be found in the relevant sections of this book; however, the commonest cause is acute otitis media.

Acute otitis media

- Antibiotic therapy is not mandatory, no major benefit being consistently demonstrated in controlled trials and spontaneous resolution being the norm. However, analgesia and antipyretic therapy are important.
- Most practitioners offer antibiotic therapy, particularly when the condition has persisted beyond 24 h, or the child looks 'toxic' (moderately or severely unwell, see Chapter 3). Such children should be observed and followed up to exclude serious complications.
- Appropriate antibiotics include amoxycillin (or co-amoxiclav) and erythromycin. The latter is preferred if *Mycoplasma* infection is suspected, or in penicillin-allergic individuals.
- Decongestants and antihistamines are of unproven value.
- All children who have had acute otitis media should ideally be reviewed at about 6 weeks to assess their hearing if there is parental concern, as some develop an effusion.
- When otitis media with effusion (glue ear) is suspected, referral for ENT audiological assessment is appropriate, usually via the general practitioner.

EAR DISCHARGE

BACKGROUND INFORMATION

- It is necessary to distinguish between the common waxy discharge of childhood and a purulent discharge.
- The causes are listed in Box 12.2.

Box 12.2 *Causes of ear discharge*

WAX

PURULENT: acute otitis media (often bloodstained)

               otitis externa

               foreign body

               chronic suppurative otitis media

CLEAR: cerebrospinal fluid

BLOOD: trauma

           foreign body

           Munchausen syndrome by proxy

DIAGNOSTIC APPROACH

History

Simple questions will usually reveal the diagnosis:

1. Is there a preceding **history of upper respiratory infection** or **trauma**?
2. **What is the discharge like** (see Box 12.2). A **smelly** discharge is *always* abnormal.
3. Is there **itch** or **discomfort**? **Itch** is usually due to otitis externa, **pain** to otitis media, although these usually occur in association in children.

Examination

- Examination of the **skin** and **external auditory canal** will often reveal **red, glazed, oedematous** skin of otitis externa (pressure over the tragus will often cause discomfort in otitis externa, whereas in chronic otitis media it will not).
- Examination of the **outer ear canal** may reveal an obvious foreign body.
- Examination of the **tympanic membrane** may reveal **central perforation**.
- **Oedematous** and **congested middle ear mucosa** (with **mucoid** or **mucopurulent discharge**) suggests *tubotympanic disease* (there may be associated **deafness**, often **unilateral**).
- A **perforation** in the **pars flaccida** (Fig. 12.1), associated with a **thin, scanty aural discharge**, and sometimes a cholesteatoma (a

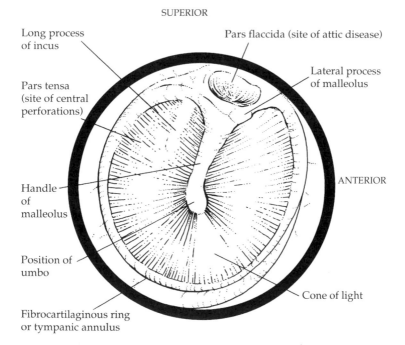

Fig. 12.1 *The right eardrum as viewed through an otoscope showing the location of landmarks.*

retraction pocket of squamous epithelium filled with debris) **visible through the perforation** suggest *atticoantral disease*.

Investigations

- **Swab** and **culture** of the discharge are important, as pathogens such as *Pseudomonas*, streptococci, staphylococci and Gram-negative organisms may be identified.
- **Radiographs** seldom influence management and do not need to be taken routinely unless **trauma** is suspected.

MANAGEMENT AND REFERRAL

- Management of a foreign body is considered in Chapter 28.
- Management of cerebrospinal fluid (CSF) leak is considered in Chapter 14. Referral for admission and antibiotic cover are important.
- Management of otitis externa:
  Topical preparations usually include a steroid (e.g. betamethasone, hydrocortisone) and antibiotic to cover the common causative organisms (e.g. gentamicin/hydrocortisone drops).
  The association with underlying otitis media in children leads many practitioners to prescribe oral broad-spectrum antibiotics, as described above.
  Advice regarding avoidance of irritants (e.g. moisture, cotton buds) is important. These are common factors in aetiology.
  Refer any cases not settling quickly to an ENT specialist (e.g. within 48 h).
- Management of other causes of purulent discharge:
  Where the clinical picture suggests *tubotympanic* disease, management is directed towards the underlying upper respiratory tract infection.
  Where the clinical picture suggests *atticoantral* disease, there is a risk of facial palsy and labyrinthine or intracranial problems: referral to an ENT specialist is mandatory.
  All other cases, or where there is diagnostic doubt, should be referred to the duty ENT specialist.

OUTCOME AND PROGNOSIS

Outcome depends upon the diagnosis. The commonest cause, otitis externa, will usually settle with the treatment outlined above, but repeated irritation or exposure to moisture occasionally causes recurrent problems.

HEARING LOSS

Hearing loss rarely presents to an A&E department, but in occasional cases it will be the sole presenting feature. It is likely to be acute in onset.

Most causes will be obvious from the history (Box 12.3). The commonest causes are wax and 'glue ear'. However, when these conditions have been excluded, urgent referral to a paediatric ENT specialist is advisable.

Box 12.3 *Causes of hearing loss*

ACQUIRED CONDITIONS

COMMON: wax
acute otitis media
otitis externa
otitis media with effusion (glue ear)
foreign body

UNCOMMON: chronic suppurative otitis media
trauma (skull fracture or direct injury)
complications of infectious diseases (e.g.
measles, meningitis)

RARE: drugs (e.g. NSAIDs, frusemide, quinine)

GENETIC CONDITIONS syndromes such as Down's,
Alport's, Pendred's etc. will not usually present to A&E

NASAL DISCHARGE

BACKGROUND INFORMATION

- A runny nose (rhinorrhea) may result from excess mucus production or nasal obstruction.
- The most common cause of a nasal discharge is a viral respiratory infection.
- Allergic rhinitis is also common, affecting 10% of all children.
- A fuller list is shown in Box 12.4.

Box 12.4 *Causes of nasal discharge*

Viral infection
Allergic rhinitis
Sinus infection
Foreign body
Adenoid hypertrophy
CSF leak

DIAGNOSTIC APPROACH

History

Most cases can be accurately diagnosed largely on history alone.

- **Clear nasal discharge** associated with **sneezing** in a **mildly unwell** child suggests a viral respiratory infection. Later in the illness, as the cold progresses and resolves, the secretions may become purulent.
- A history of **persistent nasal airway obstruction** associated with **clear rhinorrhea**, occasionally becoming very purulent (usually

with **sneezing**), suggests the possibility of allergic rhinitis. There may be a specific **event** or **environment** in which the symptoms become more apparent (suggesting possible **allergens**), or a **seasonal variation**, as with hay fever.

- **Purulent unilateral rhinorrhoea**, often **offensive** or **blood-stained**, should always suggest the possibility of a nasal foreign body (see Part V).
- **Clear unilateral rhinorrhoea**, with a history of possible **head injury**, suggests a cerebrospinal fluid (CSF) leak due to a fracture of the anterior cranial fossa.
- **Persistent nasal discharge** associated with a persistent **cough** (or recurrent cough) may suggest chronic sinus infection. Older children may complain of a feeling of being **congested**.
- A history of onset after **irritants**, such as **dust**, **dry atmosphere** and **cigarette smoke** should be sought, and might suggest vasomotor rhinitis.

Examination

Basic observations and a **general examination** should be guided by the principles outlined in Chapters 2 and 3. In most cases examination should be directed towards confirmation of the presumptive diagnosis obtained from the history. Indeed, very often the diagnosis is made on history alone.

Initial examination of the nose is best achieved in the A&E department with the use of an auroscope and (if tolerated) a nasal speculum, which should be opened vertically to avoid septal damage. Clues to diagnosis may include the following.

1. An obvious **foreign body** may be visible immediately in the nostril.
2. The **colour** and **nature** of the discharge should be confirmed, as described above.
3. Evidence of nasal obstruction should be sought by assessment of airflow using cottonwool wisps or observing the 'misting' on a cold metal spatula.
4. Evidence of **head injury** should be sought.
5. Evidence of **post-nasal** drip should be sought by examining the oropharynx.

6. Evidence of **sinus tenderness** (maxillary and frontal) should be sought by palpation.
7. As in all cases, the **ears** and **throat** should be examined thoroughly for supporting evidence and signs.
8. The **allergic salute** (rubbing the nose with the back of the hand) is a classic symptom associated with allergic rhinitis.
9. **Check the eyes** as irritation and watering may indicate an allergic periorbital cause. Any swelling, diplopia or proptosis should alert the examiner to complications of sinus infection. Urgent referral to an ENT specialist/ophthalmologist is indicated.

Investigations

- The moderately or severely unwell child should be investigated as outlined in Chapter 3.
- **Radiology** is of limited value; sinus films for fluid levels are occasionally helpful (over the age of about 6 years) if sinusitis is suspected. Occasionally a **foreign body** in the nostril may be obscured by oedema or bloodstaining and radiology may be helpful.
- Occasionally, **serum IgE levels** and **radioallergosorbent tests** (RAST) may be helpful to confirm the allergic cause of rhinitis, but not in an A&E department.

MANAGEMENT AND REFERRAL

- If a viral upper respiratory tract infection is suggested, and the child is mildly unwell, symptomatic relief is indicated with maintenance of fluid intake and **antipyretic** therapy. Decongestants are of limited value and antibiotics are required only for complications such as otitis media.
- If sinusitis is suspected **antibiotics** may be of value if there is a systemic upset or risk of complications. Decongestants such as ephedrine drops 0.25% or 0.5% given for 4–5 days can relieve the symptoms of obstruction. Antihistamines are of no proven value. Appropriate antibiotics include co-amoxiclav (50 mg kg^{-1} per 24 h in divided doses), cefaclor (40 mg kg^{-1} per 24 h in divided doses) or erythromycin in penicillin-allergic individuals. Rarely, severe complications such as septicaemia, orbital cellulitis, subdural

emphysema, brain abscess and meningitis require admission and systemic therapy.

- Surgical drainage of a sinus is rarely necessary in the uncomplicated case. It would be appropriate to review the patient in the A&E department (or GP surgery) after 48–72 h if there is no improvement.
- Allergic rhinitis may be treated with:

    1. **Removal of obvious irritant** or **allergenic** factors (easier with a cat or dog than with pollen).
    2. **Local steroids**, e.g. beclomethasone or fluticasone, applied to the nasal mucosa by insufflations are of considerable symptomatic value. Their efficacy in non-specific rhinitis is almost as marked.
    3. Oral **antihistamines** relieve associated symptoms such as eye watering, but they are less useful in relieving nasal obstruction.
    4. **Vasoconstrictors** – ephedrine 0.5% nasal drops may give symptomatic relief (for short periods only) but may lead to dependence and tachyphylaxis.
    5. **Sodium cromoglycate** (drops or spray) may be useful in nasal allergy and this is often the first choice in children, for prophylaxis 2–3 weeks before the hay fever season starts.
        Similar therapies are used (with varying success) in vasomotor rhinitis, a diagnosis made when no allergy is identified in children.

- Management of CSF leak is considered in Chapter 4 and is directed towards treatment of the head injury and **antibiotics** until rhinorrhoea resolves. Continuing discharge warrants referral to a neurosurgical unit for formal repair of the dural defect.
- Management of foreign body is considered on pages 349–351.
- All cases where the diagnosis is not obvious merit referral to an ENT specialist.

OUTCOME AND PROGNOSIS

Most cases are easily managed within the A&E department and follow-up usually falls within the realm of the GP. Prognosis depends upon diagnosis.

EPISTAXIS

BACKGROUND INFORMATION

- Nose-bleeds occur commonly in children up to 12 years old and are almost exclusively anterior, most commonly from Little's area (a plexus of vessels on the anterior–inferior portion of the nasal septum).
- Unlike adults there is no association with hypertension. Barotrauma and tumours are rare.
- The common causes are shown in Box 12.5.

Box 12.5 *Common causes of nose-bleeds*

Nasal infection (coryzal illness)
Trauma (usually nose–picking)
Foreign body
Bleeding disorders
Allergic rhinitis

DIAGNOSTIC APPROACH

The diagnosis is usually obvious, but a search for the underlying cause should be made.

History

A history of recent **trauma**, **upper respiratory illness**, **allergy** or **exposure to dry air** may be obtained. **Prolonged bleeding** or **easy bruising** in the patient or family members may provide a clue to a co-agulation disorder. An overestimate of the **amount** or **extent** of the bleeding is the norm, but the question should still be asked. Significant blood loss may be indicated by **dizziness**, **pallor** or **altered mental state** (see Chapter 21) as well as alteration of basic nursing observations.

Examination

- **Basic observations** should be recorded, and signs of shock should be sought in a general assessment. Apply first aid measures (e.g. 'pinching' the nose by applying pressure to the nasal valve area.
- Ideally, suction apparatus should be available before attempting detailed assessment of a child with epistaxis, but take a look first.
- Positioning the patient head-down will lessen the risk of aspiration if the patient is not fully conscious. A small child may be positioned on a parent's lap.
- Careful examination will often reveal the bleeding point.
- **Associated bleeding** or **lymphadenopathy** may indicate systemic disorders, and **blood under the finger nails** may be evidence of nose-picking.
- Observe closely for the presence of a **septal haematoma**, usually arising from blunt trauma to the nose.
- **Posterior bleeds** must be suspected when a source cannot be visualized.

Investigations

- Hypovolaemia should be corrected and these cases may warrant **FBC** (including platelets) and **group and saving/crossmatching** blood.
- Rarely, a **coagulation screen** may be indicated.

MANAGEMENT AND REFERRAL

- When bleeding stops spontaneously or with direct pressure (15 min continuous compression of the anterior nares between thumb and first finger) no further treatment is needed.
- Rebleeding rates are reduced if nasal vestibulitis or ulceration/crusting is treated using a barrier cream such as Naseptin or Fucidin ointment for 7–10 days.

- Continued or recurrent bleeding may need chemical cautery or electrocautery, but this would not usually be done in children without the assistance of ENT staff.
- It is uncommon for childhood epistaxis to require nasal packing and this should only be considered by ENT staff.
- Septal perforation and abscess are possible sequelae of a septal haematoma and referral is necessary for these conditions.
- Posterior bleeding must be referred to duty ENT staff.
- Beware epistaxis as part of wider facial trauma.

OUTCOME AND PROGNOSIS

Paediatric epistaxis due to local trauma is likely to recur. Preventing a nose-picking habit (e.g. by wearing gloves) is an effective intervention, and humidifiers may help in cases of dry nasal mucosa.

13 CHILDREN WITH EYE SYMPTOMS

BACKGROUND INFORMATION

- Eye injuries are more common in boys than girls by a factor of 3:1.
- In small children, time should be devoted to trying to establish a rapport with the child and gaining co-operation so that a proper examination can be made (when urgent treatment is not needed).
- If injury to the globe is obvious, tape an eye shield (or plastic cup) in place to protect the eye and refer directly.
- In the event of chemical injury, remove all solid material before irrigating the eye copiously with a stream of saline run through a giving set. In alkali burns (high pH), continue irrigation until litmus testing shows that conjunctival pH is neutral before examining the eye.
- Central neurological defects sometimes present with diplopia, proptosis, squint or visual loss of acute onset.

DIAGNOSTIC APPROACH

History

- **How** and **when** the condition developed must be established.
- In the context of injury, the nature of the **wounding agent** and its **size** and **velocity** (where appropriate) must be recorded. It is particularly important to distinguish **blunt** from potential **penetrating** trauma. Other possibilities are **radiation** or **chemical injury**.
- Eye problems of spontaneous onset are not normally serious. **Irritation**, **discharge**, **injection**, **swelling**, **epiphora** and **rhinorrhoea** are common complaints. **Diplopia** of recent onset is an important symptom which requires neurological assessment. **Blurring** or **other visual impairment** also needs to be carefully assessed.
- Record if **spectacles** are normally used.

Examination

Visual acuity must be assessed in children as in adults. Older children can be assessed using a standard Snellen chart; for smaller children, cards demonstrating shapes or objects familiar to children (such as toys) can be used for a rough assessment of vision, as can charts bearing the letter 'E' in different sizes and orientations. In small children, cover the eyes in turn while offering a toy, as occlusion of the good eye will be resisted. If acuity is impaired in older children, even with glasses, reassess using a **pin-hole** to neutralize any refractive error.

Assess the eye superficially from the outside in, documenting any abnormality of the **lids, conjunctiva, cornea** and **pupils**. This assessment is best achieved using a slit-lamp but if one is not available or the child is too small, magnification with loupes or a large lens can help.

The **upper and lower fornices** should be inspected for **foreign material** (when appropriate), but also when there is any **wound of the eyelids which may have penetrated through the underlying globe**.

Eversion of the upper lid may be resisted in children. It can sometimes be avoided by lifting the upper lid while looking from below with a strong light and asking the child to gaze inferiorly.

Inspect the anterior chambers for **haziness, blood** or **pupillary abnormality** (shape, size or response to light).

After checking for a **red reflex**, **fundoscopy** should be attempted in all children with impaired vision, a possible underlying neurological condition, or anything other than a superficial problem.

A short-acting mydriatic (e.g. tropicamide) assists fundoscopy and is not contraindicated once the pupils have been assessed, unless glaucoma is suspected.

When the condition appears superficial, **fluorescein staining** should be employed, using a blue light to assess for corneal defects. Only a small amount of fluorescein is needed (e.g. one drop, or use fluorescein-impregnated paper).

Check **external ocular movements**.

Investigations

In an A&E department, investigations are normally required only in cases of trauma:

- Radiographs should be taken if there is a possibility of penetration of the globe by a high-velocity radio-opaque object (metal or glass). This is a common problem in adults but less common in children.
- Radiographs are required when blunt injury to the facial skeleton produces swelling, bony tenderness, steps or other deformities around the orbit, or symptoms and signs of an orbital wall fracture (such as enophthalmos, diplopia, loss of upward gaze or epistaxis).
- Although immediate microscopy and Gram staining of eye swabs is rarely necessary, culture and sensitivity are useful when the cause of a conjunctivitis (bacterial, allergic or viral) is uncertain, or the condition fails to respond promptly to topical antibiotics.

Diagnosis

- Penetrating trauma may impinge directly on the eye or pass through the lids, and for this reason any lid laceration must be carefully examined for perforation, and the underlying globe inspected for lacerations which are often very subtle. In this respect, magnification is advantageous and a search should be made for small tears of the wall of the globe through which fluid or tissue appears to be herniating. The cornea and pupil may be damaged. Reduced acuity is an important sign.
- Blunt trauma is associated with bruising, swelling, bony tenderness and deformity, numbness of the cheek, surgical emphysema and epistaxis. In small children, the facial skeleton is poorly ossified and X-rays may not be helpful. The clinical diagnosis is important. Loss of upward gaze, diplopia and other abnormalities of occular movement are associated with orbital wall fractures which may produce enophthalmos. Loss of visual acuity is an important sign.
- Mild trauma commonly results from a **foreign body** on the eye or beneath the upper or lower lid.
- Corneal abrasions are associated with pain, blepharospasm and photophobia, and they take up fluorescein under blue illumination.
- Chemical injuries are usually evident from the history. It is important that the nature of the chemical is established as far as possible and advice may be sought from the Poisons Information Service.

- Another condition that should be evident from the history is **irradiation keratoconjunctivitis** associated with exposure to ultraviolet light, such as that from a sunlamp or from sunlight reflected off snow. This produces stippling of the cornea.
- Retinal detachment can be more common in children in whom the vitreous body is more adherent to the retina. Blunt trauma may therefore exert traction on the retina producing a curtain effect across the visual field, or visual disturbance resembling flashes of light or floaters.

Medical problems seen in children include **conjunctivitis** which may be bacterial, viral or allergic. Bacterial conjunctivitis is characterized by marked corneal injection and swelling with inflammation of the palpebral conjunctiva, and dried exudate on the lashes which causes the eyelids to stick together on waking. It initially involves one eye more than the other. Viral conjunctivitis (commonly adenoviral) is associated with mild upper respiratory tract infections and tends to involve one eye after the other. There is less inflammation than with bacterial conjunctivitis but irritation is a problem. Allergic conjunctivitis may be seasonal or associated with exposure to common allergens such as dust and animal fur. In more severe cases, the palpebral conjunctiva tends to form follicles.

MANAGEMENT AND REFERRAL

It may not be possible to achieve prompt co-operation from the child, and firmness with appropriate assistance may be necessary for conditions that demand immediate intervention (such as chemical exposure). In less urgent circumstances, there may be no alternative but to seek the assistance of an ophthalmologist.

The conditions listed in Box 13.1 should be referred directly to a duty ophthalmologist for attention.

An eye shield or cup should be taped over the orbit before any child with a penetrating injury to the globe is transferred. The transfer should take place with the child in the semirecumbent position.

For chemical injury, solid lumps of material should be removed before copious irrigation is performed with saline from a giving set. Alkali is one of the most noxious agents: it binds to the tissues and therefore requires irrigation for half an hour or more until the pH of the fluid in the lower fornix is neutral when tested with litmus paper. This is a painful exercise and at an early stage, the instillation of oxybuprocaine or similar local anaesthetic drops may be helpful. Sedation may also be required. After first-aid treatment, the child must be referred to an ophthalmologist if the chemical was a strong alkali, acid or other corrosive agent.

With corneal abrasions there is often blepharosphasm, and co-operation can be a problem. The early instillation of oxybuprocaine may help but an assistant is often required to hold the lids apart firmly while staining is performed with fluorescein, which will confirm the diagnosis.

Corneal abrasions are often associated with foreign bodies on the cornea or under the eyelids. These are removed as in adults, following instillation of local anaesthetic drops. However, the unco-operative child may have to be referred to the ophthalmologist. Following removal of the foreign body, the associated corneal abrasion should be treated in a standard manner with a topical antibiotic, with or without an eye-pad. Review one day later is recommended in children.

Irradiation injury is treated as in adults with an initial dose of local anaesthetic solution, supplemented by oral analgesia and padding of the eyelids for comfort.

Box 13.1 *Eye conditions to be referred to an ophthalmologist*

Lacerations involving the full thickness of the eyelid or the vicinity of the nasolacrimal duct

Penetrating injuries of the globe

Blunt trauma affecting visual acuity or producing signs of bleeding into the anterior chamber (hyphaema), disruption of the pupil or lens, or signs of a blow–out fracture

Retinal detachment

Retinal or vitreous haemorrhage

OUTCOME AND PROGNOSIS

The outcome is determined by the underlying condition, its severity and the promptness with which the eye specialist is involved.

14 CHILDREN WITH HEAD INJURIES

BACKGROUND INFORMATION

Epidemiology

Head injuries are one of the most common problems presenting to the A&E department. The commonest mechanisms of injury are road traffic accidents, bicycle accidents and falls, in that order.

Pathology

The different layers of the scalp, the skull bones, meninges, extracranial and intracranial blood vessels and the brain itself can all be injured as a direct result of the original accident (primary injury). The brain can also be damaged by the physiological and metabolic effects of the brain injury itself or by systemic injury elsewhere (secondary injury).

Primary injury to the brain at the time of the original accident can cause cerebral laceration, contusion and diffuse axonal injury (DAI).

Cerebral contusions vary in size and number. They can produce focal neurological signs. Cerebral oedema can develop around them and tentorial or foraminal herniation may result from raised intracranial pressure.

Prompt and efficient resuscitation can prevent or reduce the effects of secondary brain injury resulting from:

- Hypoxia due to an obstructed airway, chest injury or respiratory failure from whatever cause.
- Cerebral ischaemia due to hypovolaemia, shock or poor cerebral perfusion resulting from raised intracranial pressure.
- Hypoglycaemia.
- Fitting.
- Hypo- or hyperthermia.
- Development of an intracranial haematoma or cerebral oedema.

Before 18 months of age the skull sutures are unfused and the intracranial volume can easily expand without a change in intracranial pressure. The infant can thus tolerate large intracranial bleeds or cerebral oedema for longer, before neurological symptoms and signs secondary to raised intracranial pressure appear.

Trauma to the scalp causes bruising, lacerations and blood vessel injury. Lacerations can be full thickness and skull fractures can be palpated through these. Bleeding can be profuse and difficult to control.

DIAGNOSTIC APPROACH

The diagnosis of head injury may be obvious, but the injuries themselves vary from the trivial and irrelevant to the fatal. The diagnostic approach must therefore focus on the potential severity of the head injury and the associated risk.

Assessment begins with the **airway, breathing** and **circulation** (ABC) and immobilization of the cervical spine (see Chapter 23). Once these have been stabilized, determine the following.

History

- Was a significant **force** involved (e.g. a road accident or fall from a height)?
- Has there been a **loss of consciousness**?
- Is the patient **still unconscious**?
- Are there any **neurological symptoms** (including headache)?

If the answer to any of these questions is YES, a potentially severe head injury is likely. Further important points to consider are:

- **Vomiting** in the first few minutes after a head injury (even a trivial one) is common and may have been the reason the parents brought the child to hospital. Only if it persists or worsens is it likely to be an indicator of raised intracranial pressure.
- **Fits** occurring shortly after a head injury are more common than in adults. They tend to be brief, self-limiting and are only of concern if they continue, recur or are focal in nature.

- The classically described **'lucid interval'** of an extradural haematoma can continue for a long time in children before any worsening of the neurological status occurs. In the lucid interval there may not be a return to normal neurological status, only an improvement.

Examination

Bearing all the above points in mind, specific examination of the head injury and neurological status commences after the 'ABC' priorities and cervical spine immobilization.

During primary survey

1. Rapidly assess conscious level using the **AVPU** system (is the child *Alert*, responsive to *Voice*, *Pain* or *Unresponsive*?) It is a quick, reliable and easily repeatable system. The Glasgow coma scale (GCS) is used in the secondary survey (see Box 14.1).
2. Examine the **pupils** for size and reactivity to light. A sluggish response occurs before they become unequal and is thus the first ocular sign of brain injury. Unequal pupils are normally indicative of an expanding intracranial lesion, but are only of significance if the difference in pupil size is greater than 1 mm. Up to 10% of the normal population can have asymmetry of 1 mm.

During secondary survey

The detailed head to toe survey is only commenced after the primary survey and resuscitation phases are completed.

1. Examine the head by **looking** and **feeling**. The back of it can only be examined fully when the patient is 'log-rolled'. Identify **bruises** and scalp **lacerations**. Is there evidence of a penetrating injury or a depressed skull fracture? Gentle digital **palpation** of the skull through lacerations (with gloves) will help identify fractures.
2. Look specifically for signs of a base of skull fracture. This injury is rarely seen on standard skull X-rays. If it is present the patient will need a CT scan. The clues are:

- **'Raccoon' eyes**: these look like 'black eyes' which are confined to the orbital margins. They appear over a few hours.
- **Battle's sign**: bruising (with swelling) over the mastoid process.
- **Otorrhoea** or **rhinorrhoea** consisting of cerebrospinal fluid or blood. The safest approach is to assume that CSF is present in blood leaking from the nose or ear. A simple bedside test is to put a drop of the fluid on filter paper – the presence of two diffusion circles indicates that blood and CSF are both present.
- A **haemotympanum** (blood behind the tympanic membrane) or a torn eardrum. Use an auroscope to examine both ears.
- **Scleral haemorrhage** in the eye without a posterior limit. This sign is also seen in some orbital fractures. If in doubt, assume it results from a base of skull fracture.
- **Subhyaloid haemorrhage** in the fundus: this is rare and can be difficult to see with an ophthalmoscope. **Retinal haemorrhage** is also seen in non-accidental injury.

3. Assess the conscious level using the **Glasgow coma scale**. In children less than 4 years old the modified version, the children's coma scale, is used (Box 14.1). Like the AVPU system used in the primary survey, it should be repeated frequently.
4. Re-examine the **pupils** and check **vision** as transient post-traumatic blindness can occur.
5. Examine the peripheral nervous system. This does not need to be a full neurological examination, but should allow identification of **lateralizing signs** in the limbs or face. Assess motor function of the face and limbs (including tone, power, movement and reflexes). Lateralization of signs indicates an intracranial lesion. Assessment of sensation is unreliable in an unconscious patient and it can be impossible to assess cerebellar signs.
6. Frequent re-assessment of the coma scale score, pupils and motor function (known as the **mini-neurological examination**) is important, quick and detects changes early.

Box 14.1 *Glasgow coma scale and Children's coma scale*

Glasgow coma scale (4–15 years)		Children's coma scale (< 4 years)	
Response	Score	Response	Score
EYES		EYES	
Open spontaneously	4	Open spontaneously	4
Verbal command	3	React to speech	3
React to pain	2	React to pain	2
No response	1	No response	1
BEST MOTOR RESPONSE		BEST MOTOR RESPONSE	
Obeys verbal command	6	Spontaneous or obeys verbal command	6
Painful stimulus		*Painful stimulus*	
Localizes pain	5	Localizes pain	5
Flexion with pain	4	Withdraws in response to pain	4
Flexion abnormal	3	Abnormal flexion to pain	3
Extension	2	(decorticate posture)	
No response	1	Abnormal extension to pain	2
		(decerebrate posture)	
		No response	1
BEST VERBAL RESPONSE		BEST VERBAL RESPONSE	
Orientated and converses	5	Smiles, orientated to sounds, follows objects, interacts	5
Disorientated and converses	4	*Crying* (baby) *Interacts* (child)	
Inappropriate words	3	Consolable Inappropriate	4
Incomprehensible sounds	2	Inconsistently	
No response	1	consolable Moaning	3
		Inconsolable Irritable	2
		No response No response	1

The total of the score in each of the three sections is the coma scale score

Investigations

Blood

In major injury, a **full blood count**, **urea** and **electrolytes**, **glucose** testing and blood for **crossmatch** should already have been requested during the 'C' part of the Primary Survey.

Measurement of Pa_{O_2} and Pa_{CO_2} is helpful in the management of serious head injury; perform an arterial blood gas analysis in unconscious patients, and repeat it if necessary in ventilated patients.

Radiography

A **chest X-ray**, **pelvic X-ray** and a **lateral view of the cervical spine** are mandatory in multiply injured patients and should already have been obtained.

Skull radiography will identify a fracture and can also help in making decisions about discharge home from the A&E department. Request skull X-rays if there is:

- Amnesia or a loss of consciousness at any time.
- The presence of neurological symptoms or signs (i.e. significant headache, fitting or lateralizing signs, deteriorating consciousness).
- Otorrhoea or rhinorrhoea.
- Depressed skull fracture.
- Penetrating skull injury.
- Suspected foreign body.
- Significant scalp bruising or swelling.
- An accident or mechanism of injury which suggests that major forces have been involved (e.g. high-velocity accident, fall from more than 6 m).
- Difficulty in assessment (e.g. alcohol intoxication, post-ictal state, hypoglycaemia or lack of a reliable history).

Note that with increased ease of access to CT scanning, this investigation would be performed in preference to plain radiography in certain presentations.

Computerized tomography

A CT scan can be requested prior to discussion with a neurosurgeon. Some centres perform a CT scan instead of skull X-rays in a child with a coma scale score less than 12. By choosing the right scan densities and cuts, accurate information about the skull bones can be detected without an X-ray. Check the protocol in your own hospital.

- Request a CT scan after resuscitation if there is:
  a coma score less than 12
  a depressed skull fracture
  clinical evidence of a base of skull fracture or penetrating injury
  a focal neurological abnormality (fitting, lateralization)
  deteriorating conscious level (a drop of 2 points on the coma scale)
- The child should be accompanied to the scanner by an anaesthetist. The presence of a simple skull fracture alone is not an indication for a scan in a well child.

MANAGEMENT AND REFERRAL

Once the principles of airway, breathing and circulation have been addressed and resuscitation is in progress, effective treatment of hypoxia, hypovolaemia and hypoglycaemia will reduce or prevent the dangerous effects of secondary brain damage.

Secure the airway. If the coma score is 8 or less, intubation following rapid induction of anaesthesia is needed, so call for anaesthetic assistance. If the coma score is 9 or greater it may be possible to secure the airway by the use of basic airway manoeuvres or adjuncts. Do not use head tilt – anyone with significant trauma above the clavicles is at risk of having an undetected cervical spine injury. Cervical spine immobilization is established with a semirigid collar, sandbags and forehead tape until spinal X-rays and neurological tests in a fully conscious and alert child are found to be normal.

After intubation, mild hyperventilation should maintain full oxygenation and avoid hypercapnia. Advice should always be sought from neurosurgeons/anaesthetists. If the child has not been intubated and is breathing well, an oxygen mask with a reservoir bag should be applied to the face. Oxygen flow at $12 \, l \, min^{-1}$ will provide 90–95% inspired oxygen concentrations in a spontaneously breathing child.

Treat any life-threatening chest injury to maintain oxygenation and the circulation.

Hypotension from hypovolaemia underperfuses the brain. Resuscitate with fluids to a 'normal' blood pressure. Fluid overload can cause or worsen cerebral oedema. Control bleeding from scalp wounds by direct pressure with a gauze swab or a timely suture. (Hypotension resulting purely from a head injury is extremely rare. It can follow massive haemorrhage from scalp lacerations in older children or more modest scalp and/or intracranial bleeding in an infant. Before the skull sutures fuse, the intracranial volume can increase significantly as a result of oedema or haemorrhage before neurological deterioration occurs.)

Restlessness must not be attributed automatically to the head injury. Hypoxia, hypovolaemia and hypoglycaemia must be treated or excluded first. Pain, for example from a full bladder, may be the cause. Only consider a head injury to be the cause of irritability by exclusion of other factors.

Do not be scared to provide analgesia. Pain upsets the child and can increase intracranial pressure. Narcotics can be given intravenously and are safe if formulary dose schedules are followed. Regional and local anaesthetic blocks are also helpful.

Coma or worsening conscious level is a sign of raised intracranial pressure and needs to be treated promptly. The exact cause can be identified by a scan. Non-surgical treatment can begin in the resuscitation room:

- Tilt the trolley or bed to a 30° head-up position.
- After intubation, hyperventilation should be considered to maintain the Pa_{CO_2} at 3.7 kPa (28 mmHg) which requires anaesthetic assistance and monitoring of arterial blood gases.
- Consider intravenous mannitol at a dose of 0.5–1 g kg^{-1}. Neurosurgical centres have their own policies about its use so discuss the case with them first. Steroids such as dexamethasone have no place in acute head injury management.

Lateralizing or focal signs indicate an intracranial mass lesion. Do not panic. Seek neurosurgical advice as there is rarely any place for 'blind' burr-hole surgery in the resuscitation room.

Fitting in the form of a brief convulsion shortly after a minor head injury is usually of little significance. If prolonged for more than a few minutes or focal in nature then it is more sinister. After 5 min of fitting, start treatment with an anticonvulsant. Phenytoin at a loading dose of 18 mg kg^{-1} intravenously, over a 20–30 min period with ECG monitoring, is recommended (because it has no effect on the assessment of consciousness level).

Scalp lacerations are treated in a standard manner by cleaning and debridement. Closure of a wound can be performed using sutures, staples or tissue glue. A traditional method for very small and superficial wounds is to tie or glue a few strands of hair together after approximating the skin edges.

Bleeding from scalp wounds can sometimes be difficult to stop. If bleeding is not controlled by pressure or a simple suture then the vessel or vessels will have to be clipped and/or undersewn.

> ### Call for help if bleeding continues

Check tetanus status and give toxoid or immunoglobulin as indicated. There is no place for routine antibiotics in scalp wound management.

- Neurosurgical referral or consultation is required according to the same criteria as CT scanning:
  - coma score less than 12
  - depressed skull fracture
  - penetrating skull injury
  - clinical signs of a base of skull fracture
  - focal neurological signs (fitting, motor lateralization)
  - deteriorating conscious level
  - advice about the use of mannitol
- Admission for observation is indicated for:
  - confusion or any other depression of the level of consciousness
  - uncomplicated skull fracture
  - persistent neurological signs (vomiting, headache)
  - when clinical assessment is difficult (post-ictal, hypoglycaemic attack)
  - complicating medical conditions (e.g. haemophilia)
  - poor social conditions or no accompanying responsible adult

Post-traumatic amnesia with full recovery is not an indication for admission.

OUTCOME AND PROGNOSIS

Head injury is the most common single cause of death in children aged 1–15 years, accounting for 15% of deaths in this age group and 25% of deaths in the 5–15 year age group in the UK. Children less than 3 years old tend to have worse outcomes from severe head injury than older children with an equivalent injury.

Discharge home is appropriate for the majority of children attending an A&E department with a head injury. Their head injuries are minor arising from everyday falls and tumbles at home, school and play. They will have few, if any, physical signs. Scalp wounds are usually small.

- Go through the lists of indications for admission and skull X-ray as discussed above.
- If the child is well enough to be allowed home, check the social circumstances. A sensible adult (preferably a parent) should be present to observe the child. If one is not available, the child may have to be detained in the A&E department.
- A simple information sheet containing no medical jargon should be given to the carer. This should list the potential problems that may develop after a head injury and advise that the hospital or GP should be contacted if complications develop or there is any cause for concern.

15 CHILDREN WITH UPPER LIMB DYSFUNCTION

BACKGROUND INFORMATION

- Children are often brought to A&E departments with a limp arm, or one that is held across the body. They are reluctant to use the arm and passive movements are resisted. Once again, the condition may follow trauma or be of spontaneous onset.
- There are many potential causes of upper limb dysfunction, some common and others rare.
- Referred pain can occur but the presence of more than one injury in the limb may also be distracting.
- Do not hesitate to X-ray. Have a low threshold in small children, who readily sustain minor fractures.

DIAGNOSTIC APPROACH

History

- Is the child's **current or previous health** associated with any predisposition to bone, joint or other musculoskeletal problems?
- Did the problem develop as a result of known or likely (but unwitnessed) **trauma**, or is the history more indicative of **spontaneous** onset? In upper limb dysfunction, this is usually established more easily than it is in the limping child.
- **When** and **how** did the problem come to light? Slow evolution can indicate a neurological cause.

Examination

- What is the child's general **demeanour**?
- Is the child **febrile**?

- Ask the child to point to **where** it hurts.
- Ensure that the upper half of the child is completely undressed, preserving dignity as much as possible.
- At all stages, **compare** the painful limb with the normal one.
- Examine both aspects (anterior and posterior).
- In the absence of any obvious injury, assess the child's preparedness to use each major joint while gently playing with parents or carers. The normal arm usually has to be restrained when attractive objects are offered to the impaired arm.
- Briefly assess the **cervical spine**

Look

Examine the child's **posture** from the neck downwards – which joint is being held flexed or extended for comfort? Is there any **torticollis**? Look for **erythema**, **swelling**, **bruising**, **deformity**, **wasting** (suggesting an established problem) or **scarring** (from previous injury or a penetrating wound). Are the limbs symmetrical? In the upper limb, swelling is usually attributable to a fracture or to an effusion or haemarthrosis.

Feel

To gain rapport with the child, start palpation away from what you suspect to be the focal problem (e.g. opposite limb, shoulder or hand for an elbow problem). Try to distract the child and watch the facial response.

- Palpate the whole limb.
- Feel for **heat** with the back of your hand.
- Palpate the bones and soft tissues attempting to localize the **most tender area** (remember that a fracture should be tender on all aspects).
- Check the distal **circulation** and **sensation** to the best of your ability. Feel for soft tissue or bony **crepitus** on movement.

Move

Demonstrate movements you would like the child to perform, checking joints proximal or distal to the painful area first. Next, assess **active**

movements in the painful zone (note the **range**) as these will normally be more comfortable than **passive** joint movements (note the **range**). If any significant movement of a joint or bone is resisted because of pain, proceed directly to investigations (see below). Note any degree of **joint laxity**, or movements which are **more painful in some directions** than others.

You should now be coming to some conclusions concerning the likely diagnosis and this will influence your investigations.

Investigations

- Check the **temperature** and **pulse**.
- If the cause is likely to be infective or inflammatory, request a **blood count**, **differential white cell count**, **erythrocyte sedimentation rate** (ESR), **CRP** and take blood for **culture**. Consider a **sickling test** in susceptible ethnic groups.
- Request **X-rays** of specific bones or joints only if the physical signs are localized. If not, X-ray the *whole* limb. Do not hesitate to X-ray. Have a low threshold in small children who readily sustain minor fractures. Films must be taken in two or more planes.
- **Emergency microscopy** of the aspirate from inflamed superficial joints may be diagnostic.

Diagnosis

Your working diagnosis will probably be one of those listed in Box 15.1.

Box 15.1 *Diagnosis of upper limb dysfunction*

1. Fracture of clavicle, scapula, humerus, forearm, wrist or hand. The fracture may be subtle (e.g. minor buckle fracture of distal radius)

2. Septic arthritis, osteomyelitis or bone pathology (e.g. leukaemia, sarcoma)

3. Osteochondritis (e.g. of capitulum or lunate) or other overuse injury (e.g. tendinitis)

4. Shoulder, elbow or wrist sprain, pulled elbow or other soft tissue injury

5. Soft tissue infection (e.g. cellulitis, olecranon bursitis)

6. Penetrating foreign body

7. Arthropathy (e.g. viral, Henoch–Schönlein purpura, sickle-cell crisis, juvenile arthritis, rheumatic fever)

8. Pain referred from the neck, or of neurological cause

9. Loss of function of unknown cause

Fracture of the clavicle is a frequently missed diagnosis in small children. Although the injury normally heals rapidly without intervention, parents are upset when this occurs. The reasons for failing to make the diagnosis are:

- The child is not properly undressed and attention is focused on the upper arm, elbow or forearm.
- Swelling or bruising over the clavicle may be subtle in an undisplaced clavicular fracture.
- An X-ray of the upper limb may not include the medial half of the clavicle.

The *supracondylar fracture of the humerus* is one of the commonest fractures in children. Swelling is usually obvious but may be slight in undisplaced fractures, which should be suspected when tenderness is elicited over the medial and lateral supracondylar ridges. The preservation of neurovascular function is the first priority.

Forearm fractures may be subtle, especially the torus or buckle fractures of the distal radius, which is the commonest site of upper limb fracture in children. It is likely that many of these injuries are never seen in A&E departments as they heal rapidly (over about 2 weeks). Examine the cortices carefully on the X-rays. The second most common fracture is that of the supracondylar humerus, followed by those of the forearm bones.

Remember that X-rays of the whole radius and ulna including the elbow and wrist must be obtained when forearm shaft fractures are diagnosed. This is essential if a radial head dislocation associated with an ulnar shaft fracture (Monteggia fracture) or ulnar head dislocation associated with a radial shaft fracture (Galeazzi fracture) are not to be missed.

Septic arthritis of a superficial joint produces swelling, inflammation and marked tenderness in a toxic child. All movements are exquisitely painful. Blood tests and aspiration are usually confirmatory. Microscopy and Gram staining of the aspirate are emergency investigations. Radiographs are usually normal for at least 10 days.

At the elbow, an effusion is readily aspirated midway between the olecranon and lateral epicondyle (although only a few millilitres may be obtained). If inexperienced, seek assistance with aspiration of other joints.

Try to distinguish septic arthritis from less inflamed arthropathies which may affect more than one joint. Clues to the diagnosis should be obtained from a careful history and general examination.

Osteomyelitis is much less common in the upper limb but may be diagnosed from focal warmth and tenderness over bone, especially in the vicinity of a metaphysis. There may be no visible signs. A history of recent infection and a raised ESR are helpful. Radiographic changes take 10–14 days to develop but a bone scan will be positive early.

Osteochondritis in the arm usually affects the capitulum of the distal humerus or the lunate (Kienböck's disease) and results most commonly from repeated stress (e.g. bowling at cricket, gymnastics). It is diagnosed from local tenderness and increased bone density or fragmentation on X-rays.

Most *wounds or soft tissue infections* are straightforward, but in children too young to communicate well, always look for small puncture wounds and consider obtaining X-rays of the soft tissues.

Sprains in smaller children may produce no physical signs apart from mild joint tenderness, loss of function and pain on stressing the joint.

Investigations are normal. The diagnosis is often reached by excluding other conditions.

'*Pulled elbow*' is the commonest clinical diagnosis based on loss of elbow function after a traction injury, usually from a parent lifting or pulling the child (typically aged 2–8 years) by the arm. A typical traction injury may not be described in nearly half of all cases. There is loss of use but no significant elbow swelling or inflammation, and poorly localized tenderness. As the radial head is impacted into the annular ligament, X-rays normally reveal no abnormality and they should only be requested when manipulation fails (see below).

Always consider the possibility of non-accidental injury (Chapter 26).

Frequency

Pulled elbow is the most common diagnosis, followed by fractures, and finally soft tissue injuries.

MANAGEMENT

1. Fractures of the clavicle can be adequately treated by support in a broad arm sling. Humeral head, shaft and supracondylar fractures, as well as forearm fractures and dislocations, should be referred to the orthopaedic team.

    In the case of undisplaced fractures of the humerus, a high collar and cuff with or without an above-elbow backslab is appropriate. For undisplaced forearm shaft fractures, the same backslab with a sling is better. Undisplaced wrist fractures are treated with a standard Colles backslab and sling.

    Oral analgesia should be offered in all cases.

2. In possible septic arthritis, aspirate superficial joints and request immediate microscopy and Gram stain. Assistance should be sought for the aspiration of deep joints. Take blood cultures before commencing broad-spectrum anti-staphylococcal intravenous antibiotics, as recommended by orthopaedic or microbiology staff. Refer the patient to the orthopaedic team.

    In suspected osteomyelitis, refer the child to the orthopaedic team for an opinion, further investigation and treatment.

    Pathological bone conditions should be referred to a paediatrician or orthopaedic surgeon with an interest in paediatrics.

3. Osteochondritic conditions and other overuse injuries should be rested in a sling, and occasionally immobilized in plaster. They should be referred to a fracture or orthopaedic clinic.

4. Sprains disabling smaller children may need protection in an appropriate plaster cast. The injury should be reviewed 1 week later out of plaster by a senior A&E doctor. Older children may be treated like adults.

5. The pulled elbow is treated by first warning the parents that their child will suffer transient pain when the elbow is manipulated. This manoeuvre is performed with the elbow flexed to 90°, one hand gripping the child's, and the other holding the affected elbow with a thumb over the radial head. The original distraction force is reversed and the forearm is impacted into the elbow while full pronation and supination are attempted. In a typical case, pain is accompanied by a click heard and felt over the radial head. The child is then left to play for 10–15 min. *If function in the arm is not regained*, X-rays are taken. If these are normal, apply a sling and arrange for a more experienced doctor to review the injury the following day.

6. Soft tissue infections and wounds are treated as outlined in Chapter 17.

7. Deeply penetrating foreign bodies are usually difficult to remove under local anaesthesia, except in older children. Advice from senior A&E or orthopaedic staff is recommended.

8. Non-septic arthropathy should be discussed with the paediatric team.

9. For referred pain, arrange cervical X-rays and request an orthopaedic opinion.

10. A limp arm of undetermined cause (and for which all investigations are normal) should be treated as a sprain in the first instance. However, review by senior A&E staff is recommended after a day or two. A good proportion of these children spontaneously regain full use of their arm, allowing a retrospective diagnosis of sprain to be expressed with confidence.

PROGNOSIS AND OUTCOME

The outcome is generally good but clearly depends on the specific cause and pathology if present.

16 CHILDREN WITH A LIMP

BACKGROUND INFORMATION

- A child with impairment of function in the lower limb most commonly presents with a limp.
- The condition may follow trauma or be of spontaneous onset.
- The side affected is not always immediately evident but is the side on which the child spends *less* time. As a consequence, the unaffected limb takes shorter steps.
- The cause of a limp is more easily detected if it involves a superficial joint (e.g. knee).
- Bear in mind that pain from certain areas may be referred (e.g. hip pain to the knee).

DIAGNOSTIC APPROACH

History

- Is the child's **current** or **previous health** associated with any predisposition to bone, joint or other musculoskeletal problems?
- Did the problem develop as a result of known or likely (but unwitnessed) **trauma**, or is the history more indicative of **spontaneous** onset?
- **When** and **how** did the limp come to light? Prolonged evolution may indicate a neurological cause.
- Is the limp causing **pain**?
- Is the pain **diurnal**, for example worse at the start of the day (rheumatoid) or in the evening (neuromuscular)?
- Is the pain **at night**, which may indicate pain from tumours?

Examination

- What is the child's general **demeanour**?
- Is the child **febrile**?
- Ask the child to point to **where** it hurts.
- Ensure that the child is undressed to underclothes, preserving dignity as much as possible.
- At all stages, compare the painful limb with the normal one.
- Examine both aspects (anterior and posterior).
- Assess the child's **gait**, **stance** and ability to bear weight before examination on the couch. This will help to localize the source of the problem.
- Assess the **spine**.

Look

Inspect for **erythema**, **swelling**, **bruising**, **deformity** (e.g. shortening), **wasting** (suggesting an established problem) or **scarring** (from previous injury or a penetrating wound of the knee or sole). Are the buttock creases symmetrical?

Examine the child's **posture** from the spine downwards – which joint is being held flexed for comfort? Is there any **spinal** or **pelvic** (Trendelenburg) **tilt**, or lower limb **rotation**?

Feel

Start away from what you suspect to be the focal problem (e.g. opposite limb) to gain rapport with the child.

- Try to distract the child and watch the facial response.
- Feel for **heat** with the back of your hand.
- Palpate the bones and soft tissues attempting to localize the **most tender** area (remember that a fracture should be tender on all aspects).
- Check distal **circulation** and **sensation** to the best of your ability.
- Feel for soft tissue or bony **crepitus** on movement.

Move

In the older child, demonstrate movements you would like the child to perform. Start normally with spinal movement. Observe normal movements, in the company of parents, in younger children.

Check **active movements** first, which will be less painful (note the **range**). Commence **passive** joint movements away from the most painful area (note the **range**). If any significant movement of a joint or bone is resisted because of pain, proceed directly to investigations (see below). Note any degree of **joint laxity**, or movements which are **more painful in some directions** than in others.

Examine the **abdomen** if there is a possibility of referred pain (e.g. groin pain in appendicitis). Finally, perform a **neurological examination**. You should now be coming to some conclusions concerning the likely diagnosis and this will influence your investigations.

Investigations

- Check the **temperature** and **pulse**.
- If the cause is likely to be infective or inflammatory, request a **blood count**, **differential white cell count**, **ESR** and **CRP** and take blood for **culture**.
- Consider a **sickling test** in susceptible ethnic groups.
- Request **X-rays** of specific bones or joints only if the physical signs are localized. If not, X-ray the *whole* limb. Films must be taken in two or more planes. **Ultrasound** examination is helpful for hip pain if X-rays are normal.
- **Emergency microscopy** of the aspirate from inflamed superficial joints may be diagnostic.

Diagnosis

Your working diagnosis will probably be one of those listed in Box 16.1.

Box 16.1 *Diagnoses in children presenting with a limp*

1. Fracture of lumbar spine, pelvis, femur, patella, tibia or fibula, ankle or foot. This may be subtle (e.g. toddler's fracture or stress fracture)

2. Hip pain of spontaneous onset – congenital dislocation, irritable hip (1–12 yr), Perthes' disease (3–8 yr) or slipped upper femoral epiphysis (10–16 yr). The latter may follow injury

3. Septic arthritis, osteomyelitis or bone pathology (e.g. leukaemia, sarcoma)

4. Osteochondritis (avascular change, e.g. of navicular, tibial tuberosity) or overuse injury (e.g. tendinitis)

5. Knee, ankle or foot sprain, or soft tissue injury

6. Soft tissue infection (e.g. cellulitis, pre-patellar bursitis)

7. Penetrating foreign body

8. Arthropathy (e.g. viral, Henoch–Schönlein purpura, sickle-cell crisis, juvenile arthritis, rheumatic fever)

9. Pain referred from a proximal site such as the abdomen (e.g. appendix), groin (e.g. nodes, hernia) or spine (e.g. neurological)

10. Limp of unknown cause

Toddler's fracture is a term used to describe the minor buckle or torus fractures usually sustained in the leg or ankle in this age group.

Irritable hip is characterized by loss of function and moderate pain on passive movement. It often follows a mild upper respiratory tract infection. The X-rays are usually normal but there may be slight widening of the joint space by an effusion, confirmed by ultrasound scan. The diagnosis is usually made by excluding more signifcant conditions. An elevated white cell count or ESR/CRP should raise suspicion of septic arthritis or osteomyelitis. Investigations are rarely diagnostic and are usually not required if the child is clinically well, with a temperature below 38°C and no restriction of joint movement. Under these circumstances clinical review is important rather than extensive investigation.

Perthe's disease is an osteochondritis (avascular condition) of the femoral head which results in increased density, fragmentation, collapse and loss of containment of the femoral head in the acetabulum. A family history should be sought.

Slipped upper femoral epiphysis may be precipitated by obvious trauma (the 'acute' slip), it may develop more insidiously ('chronic' slip), or be aggravated by sudden stress ('acute on chronic' slip). Hip movements are painful and the slip may not be visible in the anteroposterior X-ray: a lateral Billings view is therefore essential. There is a predisposition to this condition in the unaffected hip.

Septic arthritis of a superficial joint produces a swollen, inflamed and very tender joint in a toxic child. For deep or superficial joints all movements are exquisitely painful. Blood tests and aspiration (under ultrasound control for the hip) are usually confirmatory. Microscopy and Gram staining of the aspirate are emergency investigations. The X-rays are usually normal for at least 10 days.

Try to distinguish septic arthritis from less inflamed arthropathies which may affect more than one joint. Clues to the diagnosis should be obtained from a careful history and general examination. In the presence of pus the life of articular cartilage is less than 6 h, so ask for surgical advice early.

Osteomyelitis is diagnosed from focal warmth and tenderness over bone, especially in the vicinity of a metaphysis. There may be no visible signs. A history of recent infection and a raised ESR are helpful and blood cultures may be diagnostic. Radiographic changes take 10–14 days to develop, but a bone scan will be positive early.

Osteochondritis in the foot usually affects the navicular and results most commonly from repeated stress (e.g. tap-dancing). It is diagnosed from local tenderness and increased bone density or fragmentation on X-rays. The tibial tuberosity is similarly affected in Osgood–Schlatter disease.

Most *wounds or soft tissue infections* are straightforward, but in children too young to communicate well, always examine areas such as the sole of the foot or the front of the knee for small puncture wounds, and consider obtaining X-rays of the soft tissues.

Sprains in smaller children may produce no physical signs apart from mild joint tenderness and a limp. Investigations are normal. The diagnosis is often reached by excluding other conditions.

MANAGEMENT AND REFERRAL

1. With fractures of the lumbar spine, pelvis, femur or displaced fractures of leg, ankle or foot, resuscitate the patient while excluding life-threatening injuries (e.g. hypovolaemia) by means of a primary survey (Chapter 23). Then exclude limb-threatening injury (e.g. vascular occlusion). Administer appropriate analgesia (see Chapter 25) and refer to the orthopaedic team.

   In the case of undisplaced fractures of leg, ankle or foot, apply an above-knee cast for fractures above the ankle and a below-knee cast for the ankle and foot. Prescribe oral analgesics and arrange for the limb to be elevated. Refer if the fracture is situated above the ankle.

2. Irritable hip may be treated with simple analgesia and rest at home if the child is generally well, symptoms are mild, investigations normal, the parents sensible and the patient can be reviewed the following day in A&E or by paediatric or orthopaedic staff. If this cannot be achieved, rest in hospital is best. Skin traction is rarely needed. The condition normally settles over 2–3 days.

   If Perthe's disease is a possibility, referral is indicated. The prognosis is related to the extent of femoral head involvement and the age of onset – there is less bone remodelling in older children.

   Slipped upper femoral epiphysis should be referred for an orthopaedic opinion.

3. In possible septic arthritis, aspirate superficial joints and request immediate microscopy and Gram stain. Deep joints have to be aspirated under X-ray or ultrasound control. Take blood cultures before commencing broad-spectrum antistaphylococcal intravenous antibiotics, as recommended by orthopaedic or microbiology staff. Refer the patient to the orthopaedic team.

   In suspected osteomyelitis, refer the child to the orthopaedic or paediatric team for an opinion, further investigation and treatment.

   Pathological bone conditions should be referred to a paediatrician or orthopaedic surgeon.

4. Osteochondritic conditions (e.g. Osgood–Schlatter disease) and overuse injuries may be protected in a plaster cast and referred to a fracture or orthopaedic clinic.

5. Sprains disabling smaller children may need protection in an appropriate plaster cast. The injury should be reviewed 1 week

later out of plaster by a senior A&E or orthopaedic doctor. Older children may be treated like adults.

6. Soft tissue infections and wounds are treated as outlined in Chapter 17.

7. Penetrating foreign bodies are usually difficult to remove under local anaesthesia, except in older children. Advice from senior A&E or orthopaedic staff is recommended.

8. Non-septic arthropathy should be discussed with the paediatric team.

9. For referred pain, arrange appropriate investigations and request an opinion from the relevant specialty.

10. A limp of undetermined cause (with normal investigations) should be treated as a sprain in the first instance. However, review by senior A&E staff is recommended after a day or two.

OUTCOME AND PROGNOSIS

The prognosis clearly depends on the underlying condition and there-fore varies from good with rapid recovery to poor with chronic disabil-ity. The key to optimizing the outcome is knowledge of the differential diagnosis and timely referral to senior A&E or specialist staff.

17 CHILDREN WITH WOUNDS AND SUPERFICIAL INFECTIONS

BACKGROUND INFORMATION

Compared with wounds in adults, children's wounds heal rapidly and complications are rare provided appropriate treatment is administered. When wounds are thought to warrant review in A&E, progress is best monitored by the first doctor involved.

DIAGNOSTIC APPROACH

The diagnosis is usually evident from the start. Wounds can be classified as **contusions**, **abrasions** or **lacerations** (burns are dealt with in Chapter 18).

History

- Note **when** and **how** the injury was sustained.
- Enquire whether **contamination** or the presence of **foreign material** is likely.
- Always check and record **tetanus immunization status**.
- Always consider **non-accidental injury** as a possibility, particularly when the history does not satisfactorily explain the injury.

Examination

- *Inspect* the wound noting the **situation**, **extent** and **depth** of the injury, and signs of trauma to **underlying structures** such as nerves, tendons, bone or body cavities.

- *Feel* for **heat**, to **localize tenderness**, and check **sensation** and **circulation** distally. Suspect a fracture if there is crepitus or the underlying bone is tender on all aspects.
- *Test movements*, both **active** and **passive**. The former should be less painful and will demonstrate tendon function; the latter tests bony and ligamentous integrity. Is there any soft tissue **crepitus**?

Assessment of the capillary circulation in the extremities should not be difficult, although a period of rewarming may be necessary after exposure to cold. It is, however, difficult to assess sensation in children who are too young or timid to communicate. If a nerve is at risk because of the depth and anatomical location of the wound, referral is advised and this normally ensures that the child is subjected to expert review. Remember that cutaneous nerve injury is associated with reduced sweating and skin friction (which may be tested with a plastic object – the pen test). Active movements in an unco-operative child are best assessed by a period of observation, often delegated to the parents.

In a closed limb injury, exclude signs of possible compartment syndrome (swelling over the compartment, impaired sensation in the area supplied by the compartmental nerve, persistent pain aggravated by passive stretching of compartmental muscles which is resisted).

Investigations

When indicated, **X-rays** help to define **fractures**, the extent of **contamination** with radio-opaque material (after initial wound cleansing), and the penetration of joints or body cavities by **air**. Radio-opaque debris commonly consists of glass (responsible for 5% of wounds in children) or metal (except aluminium which is not radio-opaque).

An **ultrasound** examination or **computed tomography** can assist with the diagnosis of radiolucent splinters.

MANAGEMENT AND REFERRAL

Consider **sedation** (and pain relief) for frightened or unco-operative children (see Chapter 25). The presence of the parents usually contributes towards a calm atmosphere.

Contusions

Treat contusions conservatively. Appropriate **analgesia** with encouragement to rest, apply ice, elevate and wear a supportive bandage are traditional and helpful.

Abrasions

Ensure at first presentation that the graze is fully **cleaned** to prevent tattooing by ingrained dirt, which is very difficult to rectify. It is hard to distinguish between flecks of dried blood and ingrained gravel when the wound is more than a few hours old, so prompt treatment is important.

To cleanse such an injury, the use of sponges impregnated with saline, antiseptic or hand scrub (e.g. chlorhexidine) can be recommended, in additon to moist cotton wool. Hydrogen peroxide lifts dirt off but unfortunately stings.

To reduce pain, the abrasions may be treated initially with lignocaine gel, or the child may be sedated (see Chapter 25). If the injury is extensive, infiltration of local anaesthetic solution can be worthwhile. Occasionally in small children, wound toilet under general anaesthesia is justified. Gel dressings can be helpful in loosening debris.

Abrasions are usually left exposed, or dressed if large, painful or likely otherwise to adhere to clothing. Semipermeable films do not adhere and are usually well tolerated by children.

Lacerations

Pain relief

Infiltrate with local anaesthetic solution, either as a traditional local injection or using topical cocaine and adrenaline (see p. 284), while ensuring that adequate assistance and restraint (for example, wrapping the child in a blanket) protects the patient, the injury, and the operator. Infiltration with lignocaine is less painful when a narrow needle (21 gauge or smaller) is used, pressure is applied to the skin, the injection is given slowly (e.g. over 20 s), infiltration is administered through the wound itself (unless the anaesthetic solution leaks out), and adrenaline is avoided.

Appropriate maximum dose of lignocaine is 3 mg kg^{-1} or 7 mg kg^{-1} with adrenaline (see p. 283).

Cleansing

The laceration may then be cleaned, commencing with the piecemeal removal of any gross contaminants. Standard antiseptics have not been shown to have any advantage over 0.9% saline which simply but effectively reduces bacterial density.

Cleansing depends mainly on the mechanical approach and the volume of fluid used. Pulsatile lavage, for example repeated squirting of saline from a 20 ml syringe through an 18 G needle, is effective in displacing debris from the depths of a wound. Care should be taken to avoid splashing.

Excision

Excise contused or contaminated wound margins and subcutaneous tissue (except on the hand – seek advice). The skin edges should slowly ooze blood when cut. If there is significant devitalization of skin or tissues, seek senior advice.

Exploration

Exploration of all lacerations is essential but may be difficult, even with sedation and local anaesthesia. Haemostasis, a good light, an assistant with swabs to keep the area dry, and a good set of fine instruments (skin hooks, miniature self-retaining or other retractors, Adson forceps, etc.) are important assets. Look for evidence of penetrating injury to important structures such as nerves, tendons, joints or synovial sheaths. Assume such injuries are present when the wound involves the palm. In such cases, seek the advice of more experienced staff to whom all *serious* or *problem* wounds should be referred. Do not close such a wound – decisions have to be taken before closure, even if this means that the injury has to be dressed temporarily and reassessed the following morning.

Closure

Skin closure is best delayed (delayed primary closure) in severely contaminated wounds requiring expert attention. However, in other wounds skin closure is normally achieved as in Box 17.1

Box 17.1 *Achieving skin closure.*

Suturing (record the **number of sutures**)

Glue

Adhesive strips

Hair ties on the scalp

Staples

Combinations of the above

Glue and adhesive strips must be avoided on long or moist wounds, or those under tension. Reasonable haemostasis should be achieved beforehand. With the exception of defined structures such as tendons, aponeuroses or periosteum, it is rarely necessary to stitch subcutaneous tissues.

After closure, cover the area with a minimally adherent dressing. If the area is difficult to dress (e.g. the face), leave it exposed or apply plastic spray.

Antibiotic therapy

Antiobiotic therapy is indicated for minor open fractures and penetrating wounds which may extend to joints, synovial sheaths or other important structures requiring surgical exploration. It is also recommended for:

- Lacerations of the volar aspect of the hand and fingers.
- Penetrating wounds of the sole.
- Immunocompromised states.

- Significantly contaminated wounds, for example animal or human bites.
- Wounds more than 6 h old.

Aftercare

Elevation and analgesia must not be forgotten.

For wounds that are considered uncomplicated, further care should be provided by the general practice team who should be informed of the number of sutures requiring removal and the recommended timing of this. A guide to time to removal of sutures is given in Table 17.1; more time should be allowed for wounds in areas subjected to tension.

All wounds regarded as potential problems should be reviewed in A&E. In summer, sunlight can increase pigmentation of the wound, and a barrier cream should be worn.

Table 17.1   *Timing of suture removal*

Body Area	Time to removal (days)
Face	5–6 (max.)
Scalp	7
Upper limb and front of torso	10
Lower limb and back	12

SPECIFIC WOUND TYPES

Scalp wounds

Scalp wounds may bleed profusely, requiring a temporary pressure dressing. Continued bleeding may require assistance to help locate and ligate vessels. In a small child, blood loss can be sufficient to precipitate shock (Chapter 21).

Hair should be removed from a small area around the wound. Closure is most easily obtained with hair ties and/or tissue glue. Infection occurs very rarely and antibiotics should not be necessary if appropriate wound toilet and debridement has been achieved.

Facial wounds

Small, linear wounds may close satisfactorily with adhesive strips. Tissue glue can be used away from the eyes. For larger wounds, there is no substitute for careful, anatomical closure of healthy wound margins using fine, non-absorbable monofilament material (e.g. 5/0 or 6/0 nylon). In more extensive injuries, this may necessitate general anaesthesia and referral to plastic surgeons, particularly if the vermilion border of the lips, the margin of eyelids or the nasolacrimal area is involved. Infections are rare because of the excellent blood supply, but antibiotics are advised for wounds close to the medial canthus where there is a risk of deep spread.

Tongue wounds

The tongue is easily bitten in a fall, but wounds heal very fast in this vascular tissue and no treatment is necessary in simple lacerations 1–2 cm long that are not bleeding. In smaller children, larger or pedunculated injuries should be referred for suture under general anaesthesia.

Perineal wounds

Genuine accidents can occur, for example when children fall astride the crossbar of a bicycle, but in all circumstances non-accidental causes must be considered and advice sought as appropriate. Examination of sensitive areas should be limited to that required for a decision on the need for specialist involvement. Assessment should be undertaken in a more private area of the A&E department, and care must be taken to try to retain the child's co-operation. In boys, injuries involving the genitalia may be associated with voluntary or involuntary urinary retention. In girls, the vagina may be involved. In both instances, the relevant surgical team or paediatrician should be contacted.

Wounds over joints

Always consider the possibility that wounds overlying superficial joints may have penetrated the joint capsule, posing a significant risk of septic arthritis. The knuckles are particularly susceptible, but pre-patellar injuries are common in children. The wound may also communicate with synovial sheaths or bursae.

Radiography may demonstrate air in the joint. At the knee, sterile saline injected into the suprapatellar bursa of *older* children may discharge through the wound, confirming the diagnosis.

All such injuries must be referred to the orthopaedic team for exploration, joint irrigation and closure.

Fingertip injuries

Fingertip injuries are very common in children, especially toddlers whose fingers are easily trapped in house and car doors. Fortunately, children possess powers of digital regeneration which are not enjoyed by adults. The nail is usually removed by the injury and bone may be exposed at the tip.

All such injuries should be treated conservatively in children. Any healthy pulp may be reattached with adhesive strips after both tissue surfaces have been properly cleaned. Even if the pulp becomes necrotic, it will have functioned as a temporary biological dressing and some of it may survive. Even 'non-adherent' dressings become stuck to the coagulum at the tip of the finger, so gel or antiseptic ointment dressings (and sometimes a plastic glove) are often used. Antibiotics are still recommended for open fractures of the terminal phalanx. Such injuries should be reviewed in A&E departments. Healing will take 2 weeks or more and the main challenge is removal of the dressings and strips. The dressing often has to be soaked to facilitate its removal on the first two or three visits, so frequent dressings changes are counterproductive.

Animal bites

Dogs often bite the faces of inquisitive children who approach them too closely. Such injuries cause significant family upsets. Facial wounds heal well and may be sutured by experienced persons after careful toilet and debridement to minimize scarring. Antibiotics are recommended after suturing deep wounds and they should be effective against *Pasteurella multocida* (the common pathogen – penicillin-sensitive) and *Staphylococcus aureus*. Anaerobic cover may also be required. Co-amoxiclav will be effective against all these three. In all other sites, the bite wounds which are usually small should be left open and dressed. In such circumstances the need for antibiotic treatment is controversial, but antibiotics are recommended in puncture or hand wounds which are difficult to clean. Frequent wound checks are appropriate during early healing.

Foreign bodies

Inexperienced staff should only attempt to remove foreign bodies from open wounds, not from old injuries. Even in acute injuries, assistance may be required. For metal, an image intensifier may be helpful. For complex anatomical areas (e.g. the palm), refer the child to senior staff or the appropriate surgical team unless the material is truly superficial. The younger the child, the more difficult will be the challenge, and good lighting, retraction and haemostasis are important. Set a time limit, for example 30 min, perhaps less in the younger child.

Dirty foreign bodies such as wood splinters cause persistent infections and wounds that fail to heal.

SUPERFICIAL INFECTIONS

BACKGROUND INFORMATION

There are two ends to the spectrum of infection. At one end, the child rallies against the infection and contains it, forming an abscess. At the other, the infection spreads rapidly in the form of cellulitis. Both elements may be present in a superficial infection.

DIAGNOSTIC APPROACH

History

The history may suggest localized **trauma** which can be very superficial (e.g. friction). However, there may be no **precipitating factor**.

The child's **general health** must be checked, particularly for any history of **recurrent infections**, or factors predisposing to them. Has there been a **fever**?

Examination

Examination commences with inspection which will normally reveal the classical signs of **redness**, **heat** and **swelling**. The **extent** of the inflammation is important: it may track as in typical **lymphangitis** or remain localized around an **abscess** swelling. Occasionally, purulent **discharge** will be evident. Palpation will demonstrate **tenderness** and the **distribution** of this must be recorded, particularly **proximal tenderness** or **lymphadenopathy** indicating regional spread.

Investigations

Investigations must include basic observations such as **temperature** and **pulse**, in addition to respiratory rate, capillary refill time, blood pressure, and oxygen saturation if the child is generally unwell. In the latter case, septic shock (Chapter 21) needs to be excluded and blood cultures obtained.

Occasionally, ultrasonography helps to determine the presence and extent of pus in the tissues.

MANAGEMENT AND REFERRAL

Consider **sedation** if surgical intervention in A&E is proposed.

Sometimes, it is difficult to know whether pus is present beneath an inflamed swelling or not. In such instances, attempted aspiration through a needle of reasonable calibre (19G) can help determine whether cellulitis or abscess is the correct diagnosis. The child's cooperation may be utterly lost, however. Ask for senior or surgical advice first.

Abscess

Abscesses are treated by drainage.

Small abscesses

Small abscesses in older children are amenable to **drainage** under **local anaesthesia** but some sensation often persists in the tense, inflamed, overlying skin.

- Children may not tolerate a drain, and packing may inhibit granulation tissue, need changing and increase scarring. A solution to premature closure of the aperture is the excision of a small **ellipse** of skin.
- **Microscopy and culture** of the issuing pus is not normally necessary for the majority of superficial abscesses which are caused by *Staphylococcus aureus*. Culture is recommended when any special or unusual features are present (e.g. infection following contact with animals, recurrence of a previous abscess).
- The abscess should be **washed out** with saline before being dressed.

Large abscesses

Larger abscesses, especially in small children, are best drained under general anaesthesia, so **refer** to staff in the appropriate surgical specialty.

Antibiotics are unnecessary following drainage of an abscess unless there are signs of spreading infection. Firstly, the child's defences have contained the infection which has now been expelled and continues to drain. Secondly, the thick wall of an established abscess impedes penetration of antibiotics from the circulation.

Cellulitis

For *small* areas of cellulitis, **daily review** may be undertaken in A&E after antibiotic therapy has been started. The perimeter should be delineated with a marker pen. Cellulitis is most commonly associated with streptococcal infection so the **antibiotic regimen** must be effective against these organisms (e.g. co-amoxiclav or erythromycin or penicillin *and* flucloxacillin) as well as against staphylococci. Refer children in whom cellulitis:

    is extensive

    is associated with fever (> 38°C), malaise, regional lymphadenopathy or an abscess

    occurs in infancy

    co-exists with illness or immunosuppression (e.g. steroid therapy)

18 CHILDREN WITH BURNS AND SCALDS

BACKGROUND INFORMATION

- Burn injuries in children usually generate an emotionally charged atmosphere resulting from a combination of pain in the child, guilt in the parents, and parental concern about the probability of scarring.
- Immediate or early deaths result from asphyxiation, airway compromise or extensive thermal injury. Late deaths usually occur on the intensive care unit and may be attributed to sepsis or associated organ failure. Intermediate deaths from hypovolaemia are preventable.
- All children with burns exceeding 10% of body surface area require intravascular fluid replacement.
- Burns are frequently associated with other physical injuries caused, for example, by jumping from burning buildings or the collapse of masonry.

RESUSCITATION

Airway

Immobilize the head and neck (unless other trauma can be excluded) and simultaneously open, clear and maintain the airway (see Chapter 20) while inspecting it for:

1. **Soot** in mouth, nose or sputum.
2. **Erythema** or **ulceration** from inhalation of flame.
3. **Swelling** of tongue or mucosa.
4. **Singeing** of lips, eyebrows, or face.
5. Significant **neck burns**.
6. **Stridor** or hoarseness.

In all such cases, call an anaesthetist immediately as prompt tracheal intubation is probably necessary.

Breathing

Give oxygen at high concentration (see Chapter 20) while assessing the chest. Ventilatory movement will be restricted by any full-thickness, circumferential chest burn which will require escharotomy, dividing the anaesthetic skin in both midclavicular and scapular lines with a scalpel until viable subcutaneous tissue bulges out. This rare emergency must prompt an immediate call for surgical or specialist assistance. A similar injury to the neck can obstruct the airway.

Assess respiratory function (Chapter 20) and respond to any signs of chest injury (Chapter 23). If there is evidence of **bronchospasm**, administer bronchodilator by nebulizer using oxygen.

Circulation

Assess the **circulatory status** (see Chapter 21) and establish at least one vascular access site, two in the presence of serious injury (see Chapter 23). Avoid burnt skin if possible but do not waste time. Take blood from the first cannula for **crossmatching**, **haematocrit**, **routine baseline biochemistry** and **haematology**, as well as **carboxyhaemoglobin** levels and any forensic examination that may be appropriate. **Commence infusion** with crystalloid (e.g. Hartmann's solution) but aim to change or add colloid (plasma protein fraction, albumin or synthetic colloids) as agreed with burn staff.

Assess the **percentage of body area burnt** using a combination of Wallace's 'rule of nines' and the area of the child's palm (1% of body surface) or hand and digits (1.5%). Plot the area of injury on a **Lund & Browder chart**, distinguishing simple (unblistered) erythema where possible as this should be excluded from fluid calculations.

By inspection and pin-prick, try to determine the **depth of injury** (Table 18.1) and indicate it on the chart. Assume that electrical burns or those associated with reduced consciousness (e.g. epileptic fit, drunkenness), ignition of clothing or containment within a burning building are full-thickness injuries until proved otherwise.

Table 18.1 *Depth of burn injury*

Depth of burn	Appearance	Pin-prick response
Superficial	Erythema only	Hypersensitive
		Bleeds
Superficial; partial thickness	Moist, blistered, red base	Hypersensitive
		Bleeds
Deep, partial thickness	Light pink base	Sensitive
		Bleeds
Full thickness	White, charred, leathery, waxy, dry	Insensate
		No bleeding

The child's fluid requirements are calculated from the **area of partial- and full-thickness injury**. All children with burns exceeding 10% of body surface area require intravascular fluid replacement. Use a recognized **formula** for calculating the **fluid requirement** (Box 18.1) but be prepared to add other losses (urine, vomit, etc). In serious burns, a catheter is therefore required to accurately assess urine output.

Box 18.1 *Muir & Barclay formula for calculation of fluid requirement*

COLLOID replacement needed in the first 4 hours from the time of injury:

$$\frac{\text{area (\%)} \times \text{weight (kg)}}{2} + \text{additional fluid losses}$$

If CRYSTALLOID alone is used, the volume required should be DOUBLED

This should adequately cater for the time needed to transfer the child to the burns unit

Check your calculations with staff at the burns unit and follow their recommendations

Disability (neurological) and exposure

Assess **conscious level** (AVPU) and **pupils**. Expose the whole child for examination, but be aware that children lose heat fast, particularly from burnt areas where dermal insulation is disrupted, there is hyperaemia, and plasma transudate is evaporating. Cover parts not receiving attention with dry, sterile **dressings**: cling-film or other plastic films are useful temporarily as they allow inspection without disturbance of nerve endings, and also retard evaporation. Avoid topical applications which will obscure assessment of the injury by burns unit staff.

INVESTIGATIONS AND MONITORING

- Connect a **pulse oximeter** and ECG electrodes.
- Ensure that all important **observations** are recorded (pulse, blood pressure, oxygen saturation, capillary refill, respiratory rate, etc.).
- Take blood or arrange for **blood gas tensions** to be checked.
- Request a **chest X-ray** if there is any suggestion of respiratory involvement or in trauma cases.

Secondary survey

Review the airway, breathing, and circulatory status before performing a **secondary survey** to identify other injuries (Chapter 23).

History

- Confirm the history of injury including **mechanism** and **type of burn** (hot, cold, chemical, electrical, radiation, etc.), **period of exposure** and co-existing **mechanical trauma**.
- Document any **first-aid** administered.
- Record **past** and **current** health details.

MANAGEMENT AND REFERRAL

Once resuscitation and assessment have been completed as described above, other aspects can be addressed as follows.

Neutralizing alkali with mild acid, or vice versa, tends to generate heat and is not recommended. For alkali injuries to the eye, see Chapter 13.

Electrical burns

Electrical burns are deceptive. Contact (as opposed to flash) burns produce full-thickness injuries. Current tracks selectively along neurovascular bundles and through other conducting tissues such as muscle. Beware of tissue damage some distance from the entry point, compartment syndrome and myoglobinuria. Always refer such cases for a senior opinion.

Check the **ECG**. Admit the child if:

1. There were or are any **ECG abnormalities**.
2. **Consciousness was lost**.
3. There is any history of **cardiorespiratory illness**.

OUTCOME AND PROGNOSIS

Contrary to previous belief, objective studies have not confirmed that burns produce more scarring in children than in adults.

The Collapsed Child

III

19 ABC APPROACH AND THE MANAGEMENT OF CARDIAC ARREST

- Cardiac arrest in childhood is rarely caused by primary cardiac diseases. Most cases result from respiratory depression (e.g. poisoning) or respiratory distress (e.g. asthma). Consequently, by the time of cardiac arrest the child has had a period of respiratory insufficiency, causing hypoxia, respiratory acidosis and cell damage. Other cases are secondary to circulatory failure (shock) resulting from fluid/blood loss (e.g. burns) or maldistribution (e.g. anaphylaxis) (see p. 234).
- Later chapters in this section will deal with the causes of impaired ventilation and impaired circulation. Many of the advanced techniques used in dealing with these situations are also discussed later.
- The aim of this chapter is to provide a broad outline of the techniques of paediatric basic and advanced life support. Resuscitation protocols for the common cardiac arrest situations are considered together and much of the resuscitation data are reproduced inside the front and back covers of this book.

BASIC LIFE SUPPORT TECHNIQUES

- It is essential that basic techniques are fully understood and employed effectively. Even a single rescuer can support the vital cardio-respiratory functions of a collapsed child with little or no equipment.
- The 'ABC' approach to basic life support is followed. However, the approach to a victim must be safe. The child and rescuer must be removed from danger.
- Assessment of responsiveness precedes the familiar ABC protocols. Gently shaking and asking 'are you alright' is appropriate. If trauma cannot be excluded then place one hand firmly on the forehead and shake one arm.

> If the patient is unresponsive call for help immediately

Airway

- An obstructed airway may be the main problem and airway opening manoeuvres are first employed.

> The finger sweep should not be used in children as the soft palate is easily damaged and foreign bodies may be pushed further down the airway.

- A conscious child will often find the best position to maintain the airway. An obstructed airway should be opened using the head tilt and chin lift manoeuvres (see Fig. 19.1).
- The patency of the airway is then assessed by the 'LOOK (for chest movement), LISTEN (for breath sounds) and FEEL (for breath)' techniques. The rescuer places his face above the child's, with the ear over the nose, the cheek over the mouth and the eyes looking along the line of the chest.
- The alternative airway opening technique is the jaw thrust (see Fig. 19.2). *This is the safest approach when cervical spine injury cannot be excluded.*

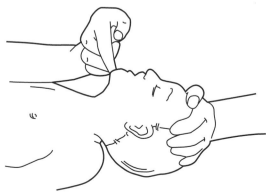

Fig. 19.1 *Head tilt/chin lift in a young child. Note: infants to neutral head position; older child 'sniffing the morning air'.*

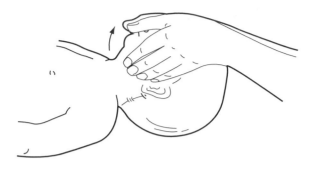

Fig. 19.2 *Jaw thrust in a child.*

- Failure of the head tilt or chin lift and jaw thrust to open the airway may raise suspicion of foreign body. Appropriate techniques for dealing with this are described later.

Breathing

- Expired air ventilation should be commenced if airway opening techniques do not result in resumption of breathing.
- Mouth to mouth (or in infants mouth to mouth and nose) ventilation should be carried out whilst maintaining an open airway. The chest should be seen to rise with slow inflations ($1-1\frac{1}{2}$ seconds per breath).
- Failure of chest expansion may indicate poor technique or obstruction (e.g. foreign body, severe asthma)
- Initially 2–5 rescue breaths should be given and subsequently the rate of breaths per min is determined by the age of the patient (see Table 19.1).

Circulation

- After the rescue breaths, attention is directed towards the circulation.
- A pulse check should be made by palpating a central pulse for up to 10 seconds. The artery chosen is usually the carotid, except in infants, in whom the brachial or femoral is easier.

Table 19.1 *Summary of basic life support techniques.*
Adapted from Nadkarni *et al.* (1997) Resuscitation vol 34, with permission

Manoeuvre	Adult and older child	Young child	Infant	Newborn	CPR/Rescue Breathing
	Older child and adult	Approximately 1–8 years of age	Less than 1 year of age	Less than 1 month (neonate)	Check responsiveness Open airway Activate emergency medical services as soon as feasible
Airway	Head tilt-chin lift (if trauma use jaw thrust)	Head tilt-chin lift (if trauma use jaw thrust)	Head tilt-chin lift (if trauma use jaw thrust)	Head tilt-chin lift (if trauma use jaw thrust)	
Breathing Initial	2–5 breaths at approximately $1\frac{1}{2}$ s per breath	2–5 breaths at approximately $1\frac{1}{2}$ s per breath	2–5 breaths at approximately $1\frac{1}{2}$ s per breath	2–5 breaths at approximately $1\frac{1}{2}$ s per breath	CHECK BREATHING If victim breathing: Place in recovery position If no chest rise: reposition and reattempt up to 5 times
Subsequent	12 breaths min^{-1} (approximately)	20 breaths min^{-1} (approximately)	20 breaths min^{-1} (approximately)	30–60 breaths min^{-1} (approximately)	
Foreign body airway obstruction	Abdominal thrusts or back blows	Abdominal thrusts or back blows or chest thrusts	Abdominal thrusts or chest thrusts (No abdominal thrusts or back blows)	Suction (No abdominal thrusts	
Circulation Pulse check	Carotid	Carotid	Brachial	Umbilical (newborn only)	ASSESS FOR SIGNS OF LIFE *If pulse present but breathing absent:* provide rescue breaths *If pulse not confiidentl felt or 60 min^{-1} and poor perfusion:* chest compressions
Compression landmarks	Lower half of sternum	Lower half of sternum	One fiinger width below inter mammary line	One fiinger width below inter mammary line	
Compression method	Heel of one hand, other hand on top	Heel of one hand	Two or three fiinger	Two fiingers or encircling thumbs	
Compression depth	Approximately 1/3 the depth of the chest	Approximately 1/3 the depth of the chest	Approximately 1/3 the depth of the chest	Approximately 1/3 the depth of the chest	Continue BLS: Integrate procedures appropriate for new born, paediatric or adult advanced life support at earliest opportunity
Compression rate	Approximately 100 min^{-1}	Approximately 100 min^{-1}	Approximately 100 min^{-1}	Approximately 120 min^{-1}	
Compression/ ventilation ratio	15:2 (single rescuer) 5:1 (two rescuers)	5:1	5:1	3:1	

- If the pulse is slow (rate < 60 min) or absent, chest compression must be commenced.
- Compression techniques, rate, and ventilation/compression ratios all vary according to the size of the patient and details are summarized in Table 19.1 and Fig. 19.4.

CHOKING

If the onset of respiratory distress is sudden and associated with coughing, stridor or gagging, a foreign body may be suspected. Physical methods of clearing the airway are described below but

> Do not use these methods if the cause of the obstruction is unclear unless there is severe increasing dyspnoea or complete apnoea

Techniques:

1. Back blows:
   - a baby may be placed along one of the rescuers arms in a 'head down' position, the rescuers arm then being placed along the thigh. Five back blows are delivered between the scapulae with the freehand (see Fig. 19.3a)
   - a small child may be rested across a rescuer's lap and the same technique used (see Fig. 19.3b).

2. Chest thrusts:
   - a baby should be placed along the rescuers thigh, in the manner described above, but this time supine. Five chest thrusts are given over the landmark for cardiac compression but at a slower rate (see Fig. 19.5)
   - a small child may be reclined on a rescuers lap and the same technique is used

3. Heimlich manoeuvre:

> This technique must not be used in infants as it may cause intra abdominal injury

- In the Heimlich manoeuvre the abdomen is grasped from behind with a fist covered with a hand and a sharp upwards squeeze in the subdiaphramatic area is given. This technique can be applied in the supine patient using the heel of a hand.

(a)

(b)

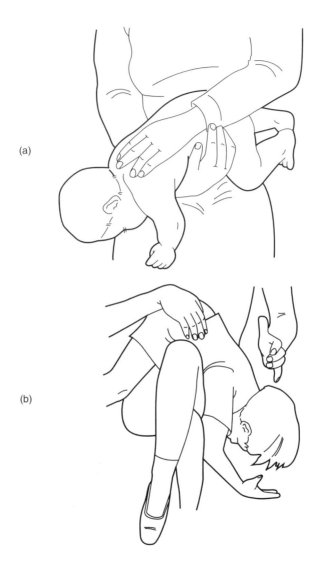

Fig. 19.3a and b *Techniques for use in a choking child.*

- If all the above techniques are unsuccessful and there is no air movement, direct laryngoscopy should be attempted to see if the foreign body is removable with Magill's forceps; emergency crico-thyrotomy may be necessary.

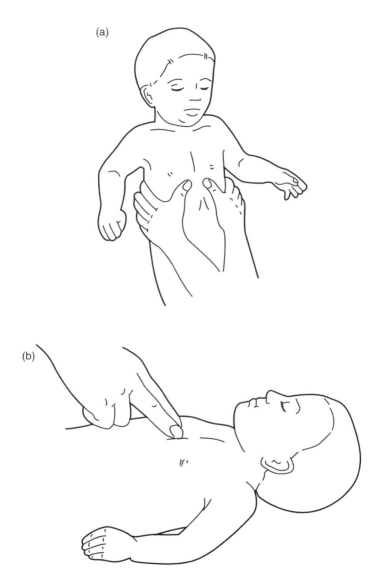

Fig. 19.4 a and b *Chest compression (see text).*

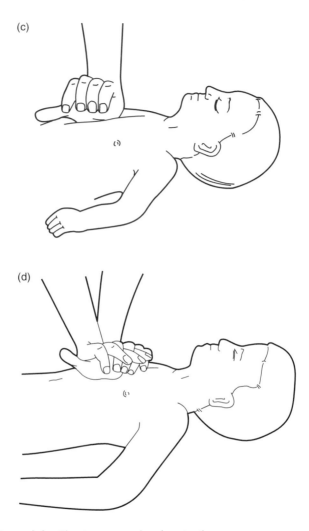

Fig. 19.4 c and d *Chest compression (see text).*

ADVANCED LIFE SUPPORT TECHNIQUES:

- Advanced life support of the airway and ventilation are described in Chapters 20 and 21.

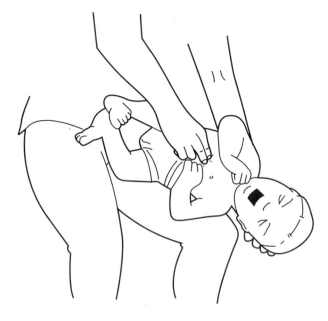

Fig. 19.5 *Technique for use in a choking child.*

Management of cardiac arrest

Cardiac arrest is the absence of a major pulse in the unresponsive child. Three cardiac arrest rhythms exist:

1. Asystole
2. Ventricular fibrillation
3. Electromechanical dissociation

Asystole

This is the commonest arrhythmia in pulseless children and because it is the response to prolonged severe hypoxia and acidosis it is often associated with a poor outcome. The ECG appearance (see Fig. 19.6) is almost a straight line but care must be taken to exclude technical problems (e.g. disconnected leads or low gain). Management is according to the flow diagram (Fig. 19.7)

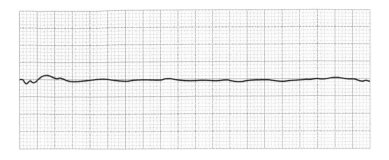

Fig. 19.6 *Asystole.*

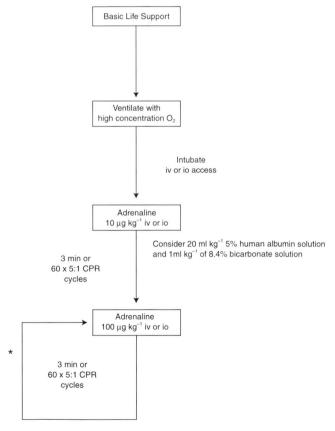

Fig. 19.7 *Management of asystole. *Consider a continuous infusion of adrenaline (2 µg kg^{-1} min^{-1}). Note: calcium should only be used if there is evidence of hypocalcaemia, hyperkalaemia or hypermagnesaemia.*

Ventricular fibrillation (VF)

VF (Fig. 19.8) is uncommon in childhood but can occur in cases of poisoning (particularly involving tricyclic antidepressants), those with cardiac disease and secondary to electrolyte disturbance or hypothermia.

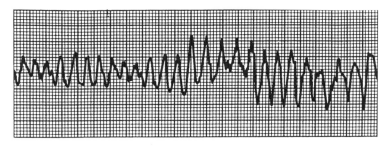

Fig. 19.8   *Ventricular fibrillation.*

Management is depicted in the flow diagram. (Fig. 19.9)

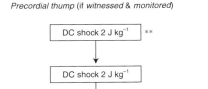
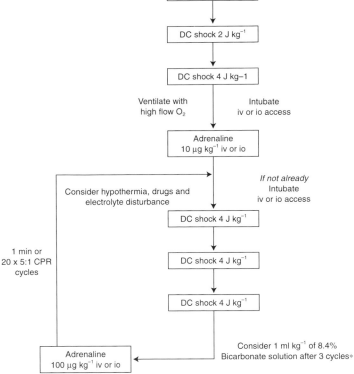

Precordial thump (if *witnessed* & *monitored*)

DC shock 2 J kg^{-1} **

DC shock 2 J kg^{-1}

DC shock 4 J kg-1

Ventilate with high flow O$_2$ | Intubate iv or io access

Adrenaline 10 µg kg^{-1} iv or io

If not already Intubate iv or io access

Consider hypothermia, drugs and electrolyte disturbance

DC shock 4 J kg^{-1}

1 min or 20 x 5:1 CPR cycles

DC shock 4 J kg^{-1}

DC shock 4 J kg^{-1}

Consider 1 ml kg^{-1} of 8.4% Bicarbonate solution after 3 cycles*

Adrenaline 100 µg kg^{-1} iv or io

Fig. 19.9 *Management of ventricular fibrillation. *Lignocaine 1 mg kg^{-1} iv/io can also be considered after 3 cycles. ** Paediatric paddles should be used for children under 10 kg (one electrode at the apex, one electrode to the right of the sternum below the clavicle). If only adult paddles are available, one may be placed on infant's back and the other over the left lower part of the chest at the front.*

Electromechanical dissociation (EMD)

This is the presence of recognisable QRS complexes on the ECG monitor in association with the absence of a palpable pulse, usually as a consequence of shock (see Chapter 21). Management is shown in the flow diagram (Fig. 19.10).

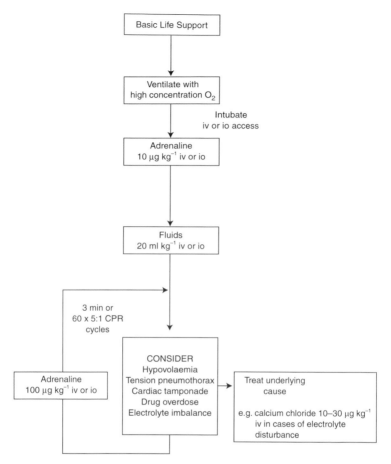

Fig. 19.10 *Management of electromechanical dissociation.*

POST-RESUSCITATION MANAGEMENT

The basic aim in post-resuscitation management is the prevention of multisystem failure in the hours following resuscitation. The following is a guide only and senior help should always be sought.

1. All children need to be monitored for:
   pulse rate/rhythm
   Sao_2

        temperature
        blood pressure
        urine output
        arterial pH and gases (ABGs)
        (preferably) end tidal CO_2 monitoring

2. Investigations following successful resuscitation include:
        chest X-ray
        ECG
        full blood count
        group and save serum
        clotting screen
        blood glucose
        liver function tests
        urea and electrolytes

3. Children with impaired consciousness or a depressed gag reflex should remain intubated and ventilated to maintain $Sao_2 \geq 95\%$ and ABGs normal.

4. Poor cardiac output needs to be addressed as there may be a need for further circulatory expansion, inotropic drug support or vasodilators. Post resuscitation arrhythmias (see page 205) may need to be treated.

5. Care should be taken to avoid hypothermia (cover with blankets and use warmed fluids) and hypoglycaemia (correct with 10% dextrose)

STOPPING RESUSCITATION ATTEMPTS

The team leader of a resuscitation team, usually a senior member of A&E or paediatric staff, will ultimately have to make the difficult decision of when to stop an apparently unsuccessful resuscitation attempt. No evidence of cardiovascular improvement or cerebral activity despite 30 min of CPR is usually taken to be an indication that further attempts are futile, the exception being the care of the hypothermic child (in whom resuscitation must continue until the patient has a core temperature of at least 32°C)

MANAGEMENT OF COMMON ARRHYTHMIAS

The following section is written as a guide only and in all cases advice should be sought from senior A&E or paediatric staff.

SINUS TACHYCARDIA:

Causes: fever, dehydration, illness

Presentation: as the underlying illness

Appearance: see Fig. 19.11: regular QRS complexes all equal, each preceded by a *p* wave; rate can be up to 220 min^{-1} in infants

Treatment: treat the underlying cause

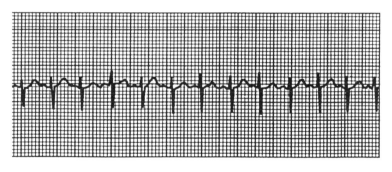

Fig. 19.11 *Sinus tachycardia*

SUPRAVENTRICULAR TACHYCARDIA:

Causes: the most common cardiac arrhythmia in infancy and childhood; aberrant conduction pathways

Presentation: poor feeding, sweating, poor colour, hepatomegaly, signs of cardiac failure, collapse

Appearance: see Fig 19.12; narrow regular QRS complexes; rate over 220 min^{-1} and up to 300 min^{-1}

Treatment: If shocked: synchronous DC cardioversion 0.5 J kg^{-1}– 1 J kg^{-1}, increasing to 2 J kg^{-1} if ineffective.

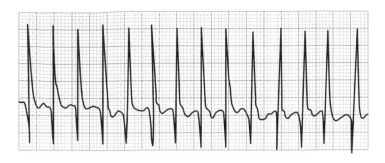

Fig. 19.12 *Supraventricular tachycardia*

If no shock:

1. Try vagal stimulation e.g. diving reflex (i.e. immersion of an infant into iced water for about 5 s); one sided carotid massage; or the Valsalva manoeuvre (in older children)
2. Consider intravenous adenosine, initially at a dose of 50 µg kg^{-1} iv, increasing to 100 µg kg^{-1} after 2 min if not successful. A further dose of 250 µg kg^{-1} may be given. Adenosine has a half life of only 10 s but has well recognised side-effects (e.g. nausea, chest tightness)

VENTRICULAR TACHYCARDIA:

Causes: uncommon in childhood, usually secondary to cardio-myopathy or following cardiac arrest, poisoning or electrolyte disturbance. May occur in children with congenital heart disease

Presentation: patients usually present in a state of circulatory collapse with poor tissue perfusion and the rhythm may degenerate into VF

Appearance: see Fig. 19.13: defined as 3 or more ectopic ventricular beats and considered sustained if continuing longer than 30 s. Ventricular rate 120–250 min^{-1}. Wide QRS complexes.

Treatment: If shocked: non synchronous DC shock 0.5–1 J kg^{-1},

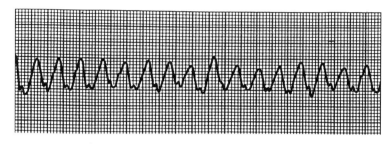

Fig. 19.13 *Ventricular tachycardia*

increasing to 2 J kg^{-1} if ineffective. Consider a bolus/ infusion of lignocaine

If no shock: lignocaine 0.5–1 mg kg^{-1} iv as a bolus, followed by infusion at 10–50 µg kg^{-1} min^{-1}. Alternatives include amiodarone and phenytoin.

BRADYCARDIA:

Causes: Often a response to profound hypoxia and acidosis; secondary to systemic illness and increased intracranial pressure; during tracheal intubation; occasionally in fit adolescents

Presentation: Dependent on underlying cause but there may be no symptoms.

Appearance: Fig. 19.14

Treatment: If shocked: treat underlying hypoxia and shock (see Chapter 21) then consider adrenaline (10 µg kg^{-1}) and atropine (20 µg kg^{-1})

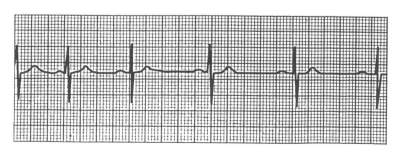

Fig. 19.14 *Sinus bradycardia during suctioning*

20 AIRWAY AND BREATHING PROBLEMS

BACKGROUND INFORMATION

- Children have a more rapid circulation and more rapid respiratory rate than adults. The smaller the child the more pronounced the difference (see Part VI).

- In childhood primary respiratory failure is a more common cause of death than cardiac arrest as the heart is normally healthy. Failure to prevent or treat respiratory arrest may cause a secondary cardiac arrest from which an uncomplicated recovery is unlikely.

- Respiratory failure in a young patient can be viewed as a failure to meet the body's oxygen demand. Very high Pa_{CO_2} levels will produce significant respiratory acidosis and depression of conscious level.

- Biochemically, a good rule of thumb is that respiratory failure has occurred when the Pa_{CO_2} is more than 60 mmHg (8 kPa). However, neonates usually have a lower plasma pH and a lower Pa_{O_2} (70 mmHg, 9.3 kPa) than older children or adults, while the Pa_{CO_2} is similar (35–45 mmHg, 4.7–6 kPa).

- Although strictly speaking a Pa_{CO_2} of 50 mmHg (6.7 kPa), implies respiratory failure, it is the combination of a fall in Pa_{O_2} and a rise in Pa_{CO_2} which is significant. The value serves as a trend and guide to management in the A&E department. The aim is to recognize impending respiratory failure and treat it early. Causes of impaired ventilation are listed in Box 20.1. In children both anatomical and physiological differences may contribute to the respiratory failure.

Box 20.1 *Causes of impaired ventilation*

Upper airway problems

Lower airway problems

Lung disorders

Extrapulmonary causes

Neuromuscular disorders

Neurogenic causes

Anatomical differences

- The larynx is more conically shaped in small children.
- The larynx lies higher in the neck than in the adult (i.e. opposite the fourth and fifth cervical vertebrae).
- The narrowest point in the small child's airway is the cricoid cartilage which takes the form of a complete ring encircling the upper end of the trachea.

> **The vocal cords are not the narrowest part of the airway in small children**

- As the child grows, the cricoid cartilage increases in diameter faster than the trachea and at about 8 years of age the proportions are roughly the same as in the adult.
- The larynx of an infant or small child is particularly susceptible to oedema which may severely narrow the airway, even after mild trauma or infection. This increases airway resistance and the work of breathing. The upper airway may be further narrowed by large tonsils or adenoids.
- The bronchi and bronchioles have a small cross-sectional area compared with those of adults and are much more easily occluded by oedema and secretions.

Physiological differences

- Chest wall compliance is very high in small children. Attempts to generate high negative intrathoracic pressures to overcome substantial airway resistance results in marked intercostal and subcostal **recession**.
- The respiratory muscles are weak in small children and breathing is largely diaphragmatic under the age of 2 years. Inspiratory efforts to overcome increased resistance result in a much increased **work of breathing**, and respiratory muscle fatigue develops rapidly leading to respiratory failure, or **apnoea** in small babies.
- Babies up to 6 weeks old are obligate nasal breathers.
- In neonates the functional residual capacity is established in the first few breaths. The functional residual capacity as a proportion of lung volume is initially low but it increases throughout infancy. In smaller children, the small airways close at a lung volume (closing volume) which is within the tidal range of breathing. This makes babies and small infants prone to distal airway collapse when the airways are narrowed by infection.
- Infants have a high metabolic rate and oxygen requirement resulting in a **respiratory rate** of 30 min^{-1} or more in the first year of life (see Part VI).

Congenital problems such as tracheo-oesophageal fistula are usually apparent at or soon after birth and they therefore present rarely to the A&E department. However, vascular rings, tracheomalacia, laryngeal webs, nerve palsies and tumours can manifest themselves at a later stage.

The most common reason for breathing difficulty in a young child presenting to the A&E department is a respiratory infection such as croup, epiglottitis and bronchiolitis or asthma. These conditions are described in Chapter 6.

DIAGNOSTIC APPROACH

History

- Upper airway problems (e.g. croup and epiglottitis) can often be distinguished from lower airway problems (asthma, bronchiolitis) by history alone.

Table 20.1 *Checklist for questions*

Symptom	Questions

Feels unwell	Is the child
	    eating?
	    drinking?
	    feverish? (high in epiglottitis, tracheitis, moderate in croup)
	    vomiting?

Tachypnoea	Congenital heart disease? Asthma?
Breathlessness	At rest? With exercise – how much? Too breathless to walk? Waking the child from sleep? Cannot sleep? Cannot lie flat?
Cough	Paroxysmal? (pertussis) Barking? (croup) Wheezy? (asthma, brochiolitis)
Stridor	Inspiratory? Expiratory? Accompanied by recession?
Hoarse voice or lost voice, cannot drink, drooling	Can child swallow? Toxic?
Cyanosis	Heart disease?
Pleuritic or abdominal pain	Sputum? (*Note*: all small children swallow sputum) Colour of sputum? Blood in sputum?

- A symptom-based approach is helpful (see Chapter 6). Most children with any significant respiratory infection feel unwell, refuse to eat and drink, and have a fever which may be very high (e.g. acute epiglottitis). Table 20.1 may be useful as a checklist for questions.

Examination

> In a severely ill child with respiratory compromise:
> call for senior A&E/anaesthetic help and
> do not distress the child as this may precipitate respiratory failure.

- A child who is active is probably not too unwell.
- In severe cases, only a visual examination may be possible since the gentlest examination, even listening to the chest, may precipitate complete airway obstruction. Useful findings which may be observed without distressing the child are detailed in Chapters 2, 3 and 6 and include:

  prominent accessory muscles, nasal flaring, and **intercostal or sternal recession** indicating significant respiratory difficulty and increased work of breathing

  tachypnoea

  cyanosis – an ominous sign in children

- A gentle examination of the child may be possible looking for cardiac signs including:

  tachycardia

  gallop rhythm

  hepatosplenomegaly

  oedema

  raised jugular venous pressure (JVP)

When there is a history of congenital heart disease, respiratory rather than cardiac failure is more likely. Children with primary heart disease may present in respiratory failure and decompensate more quickly.

- The major contraindication to physical examination is acute epiglottitis. This diagnosis *must* be made on history alone since the gentlest examination can pecipitate airway obstruction.

> On no account must the throat be examined in epiglottitis
> except under general anaesthesia

MANAGEMENT AND REFERRAL

For children with impending respiratory failure, assessment and management are carried out simultaneously by giving **oxygen** and **calling for senior help**. Severe upper airway obstruction and life-threatening asthma call for prompt and effective action. Management of individual conditions has been considered in Chapter 6. However, the initial management of respiratory emergencies in the A&E department is summarized below for convenience:

Initial management

Acute epiglottitis

If possible, nothing should be done to disturb the child until the anaesthetist arrives. If the child is obtunded, high-flow **oxygen** should be given. Airway opening manoeuvres may have to be applied if complete airway obstruction occurs (see below). Intubation should not be attempted by unskilled staff unless cardio-respiratory arrest has occurred.

Croup

If there is respiratory distress give **oxygen** by face mask, preferably **humidified**. **Nebulized budesonide** (2 mg) has been shown to be effective in reducing the severity of croup. It should be given with oxygen and administered to all but mild cases of croup. The onset of action is gradual (after about 30 min) and may last up to 12 h. Some practitioners use oral steroids.

   Nebulized adrenaline 5 mg (5 ml of 1:1000) should be given to *severe* cases at any age. This is thought to work by decreasing mucosal oedema. An **ECG** and **oxygen saturation monitoring** are required. A transient tachycardia may occur (but arrhythmias are very rare. A 'rebound' worsening may also occur). Adrenaline buys time to obtain skilled help and transfer the child to a high-dependency area. If this treatment proves ineffective and respiratory failure is impending, urgent tracheal intubation may be required.

Steam is often advocated for the domiciliary treatment of mild cases of croup but it has no place in the management of moderate or severe cases. However, dry gases must be adequately humidified.

Tracheal intubation should only be performed by those skilled in the technique as a tube several sizes smaller than anticipated may be required. Intubation is indicated if the child is becoming exhausted and the tube may have to remain in place for up to 14 days until the mucosal swelling resolves.

Acute severe asthma

> Remember, acute asthma may be mimicked by an inhaled foreign body, bronchiolitis, epiglottitis or croup

In addition to the clinical signs, the best indicators of severity are **oxygen saturation** and **peak expiratory flow rate**. If the peak flow rate is less than 40% of that predicted or **breath sounds are virtually inaudible**, respiratory arrest is imminent. **Clouding of consciousnes** reflects hypoxia and hypercarbia and demands immediate treatment.

Full details of the suggested protocol for the assessment of a child with asthma can be found on page 47. The sequence of treatment for imminent respiratory failure from acute asthma is restated in Box 20.2 for convenience.

Box 20.2 *Treatment sequence for imminent respiratory failure in asthma*

---

1.   Nebulized salbutamol 2.5–5 mg in oxygen (not air), repeated as necessary *Continue O_2 therapy at all times.*

2(i).   Intravenous aminophylline 5 mg kg^{-1} if no response to nebulized salbutamol after 10–15 minutes or Sao_2 remains less than 85% (OMIT IF CHILD IS ALREADY RECEIVING THEOPHYLLINES)

(ii).   Consider aminophylline infusion 1 mg kg^{-1} h^{-1}

(iii).   Intravenous steroids: hydrocortisone 4 mg kg^{-1} followed by 1 mg kg^{-1} h^{-1}

3.   Consider nebulized ipratropium 250 µg in oxygen

4.   Artificial ventilation if respiratory failure persists as the child will be exhausted (see page 219 for indications to ventilate). See p. 47, Fig. 6.1.

5.   Check blood glucose level in exhausted children and initiate treatment for dehydration, but avoid fluid overload

6.   Admit promptly to the intensive care unit

Bronchiolitis

The assessment and management of bronchiolitis is considered in Chapter 6. The most severe problems occur in infants with a history of **prematurity**, **chronic lung disease** or **congenital heart disease**. The risk of sudden apnoea is high in neonates. Treatment is directed towards reducing the work of breathing. Saturation monitoring is mandatory. Apnoeic attacks can be safely managed with bag and mask ventilation until the anaesthetist arrives. Severe cases will require mechanical ventilation and such children should be transferred urgently to the intensive care unit. When available, humidified oxygen should be provided through a head box and adequate hydration and nutrition should be maintained.

Inhaled foreign body

Give high-flow oxygen by mask if the child is still breathing, but life-threatening apnoea may occur either reflexly or from mechanical obstruction or laryngeal spasm.

If the child is unconscious, call urgently for an anaesthetist and an ENT surgeon and examine the pharynx with a laryngoscope. A visible foreign body can be removed with Magill forceps. Avoid finger-sweeps in small children.

In the absence of specialist skills, apply chest thrusts in the infant or abdominal thrusts in the older child. In the apnoeic child, bag and mask ventilation can force the foreign body into a main bronchus allowing the other lung to be ventilated.

Cricothyrotomy may be required (see Part VI).

Seconds count!

Advanced respiratory life support techniques

All doctors working in A&E departments should attempt to acquire life support skills and ensure they are familiar with the equipment in their own department.

Ventilation can be assisted even in semiconscious individuals.

Airways

- An oropharyngeal airway may help to relieve obstruction but often fails to overcome it completely because of the loss of laryngeal and pharyngeal muscle tone in the unconscious child.

   The disposable plastic airways used nowadays are based on the Guedel airway but are usually not quite curved enough to hold forward the large tongue of a small child. Airways are manufactured in sizes 000, 00, 0, 1, 1a, 2, 3 and 4. Size 1a is most useful for infants.
- Nasal airways are made of soft silicone rubber, red rubber or soft plastic, but their use in younger children may cause trauma to the nasal cavity and substantial bleeding from the adenoids.
- Assessing airway size:
   1. An oral airway should cover the distance from the angle of the jaw to the midpoint of the chin.
   2. A nasal airway should correspond to the distance between the tip of the nose and the tragus of the ear and have a diameter similar to that of the child's little finger.

- Only attempt to insert an airway in an unconscious patient. If reflexes are present, severe laryngospasm, bradycardia or vomiting may occur.
- The oral airway is inserted by depressing the tongue with a laryngoscope blade or spatula in infants, or by inserting it at first inverted and then rotating it over the tongue in older children.
- The nasal airway should pass easily through the nostril and then be inserted perpendicular to the face. Use only gentle pressure as it is easy to traumatize the nasal passage and adenoids.

Bag and mask ventilation

- Self-inflating bags are manufactured in various sizes. A capacity of 500 ml is suitable for small children (< 5 years) including babies, and the adult size is appropriate for all other age groups.

- Self-inflating bags for infants have a 'pop-off' valve set to open at about 20 cm H_2O. However, pressures in excess of this are frequently required to ventilate the lungs in children with respiratory disease and the valve must be overridden. It is virtually impossible to generate enough pressure with a self-inflating bag to damage the lungs.
- All resuscitation bags must be fitted with a reservoir for oxygen, otherwise high concentrations cannot be delivered. The valve assembly must not be capable of reverse assembly and should be regularly checked. The whole unit must be autoclavable or disposable.
- The contoured face masks supplied sometimes have pneumatic or foam cushions to effect a seal on the face, but in small children the best seal is often obtained with a round face mask or a Rendell–Baker–Soucek anaesthetic face mask. Some practice is required with the latter to produce a good seal.
- Pressure should only be applied to bony structures and care must be taken to avoid pressing on the soft tissues beneath the chin, which will force the tongue up into the airway.
- Small infants should be ventilated at the rate of 30 min^{-1} or more, children from 5–10 years at 20–25 min^{-1} and adolescents at 15–20 min^{-1} with sufficient tidal volume to produce chest expansion. Unless this is achieved, hypercarbia will occur. Ventilation is more efficient in intubated patients.

Laryngeal mask airway

The laryngeal mask airway (LMA) has an established place in anaesthetic practice and may enable the child to be ventilated when the use of a face mask is impractical and tracheal intubation cannot be achieved. The LMA is only to be used by those with the necessary experience.

> **On no account should a laryngeal mask airway be used without formal training**

- The LMA can be placed in the unconscious patient even when muscle tone prevents adequate laryngoscopy.
- Insertion may cause coughing or rejection which indicates that the procedure should be abandoned.
- The LMA does not always guarantee an unobstructed airway.
- There are four sizes suitable for use in children; those manufactured with armoured tubing are more difficult to insert.

Breathing circuits

- Anaesthetic breathing circuits are usually preferred by anaesthetists because 100% oxygen can be given. A self-inflating bag with a reservoir can approach only 90% oxygen. With practice, circuits are easy to use, but using the T-piece requires considerable skill to maintain the open-tailed bag full while ventilating the patient. Furthermore, a knowledge of the correct gas flows is required (not less that $3\,l\,min^{-1}$ in babies, $6\,l\,min^{-1}$ in teenagers).
- The circuits must be readily available to experienced anaesthetic personnel working in the A&E department.

Tracheal intubation

- Some skill in tracheal intubation should be acquired by all doctors working in A&E departments.
- A range of tracheal tubes must be available in all resuscitation areas.
- Formulae have been devised to estimate the length and internal diameter appropriate to the average child (see p. 364 or Box 20.3).
- Tube sizes are better related to age than weight, but exceptionally large or small children may need one size above or below the average for their age.

- The larynx in small children is higher in the neck, more anterior and covered by a large U-shaped epiglottis.
- Uncuffed tubes are used if the internal diameter is less than 6.5 mm (8 years of age).
- Tube connectors may vary. The ISO standard is 15 mm and is widely available; 8.5 mm connectors are often preferred for babies in the operating theatre. Many types of older metal connectors can still be found.

> **It is vital to ensure that everything fits before use and familiarity with equipment available within the department is of paramount importance**

Indications

1. Maintenance of the difficult airway.
2. Inadequate ventilation by bag and mask.
3. Risk of regurgitation and aspiration.
4. Transport to another centre (if airway compromised).
5. Flail chest.
6. Facial and airway burns.
7. Major trauma.
8. Cardiorespiratory arrest.

Relative contraindications

1. Not every patient with breathing difficulties needs to be intubated; *adequate oxygenation* is the aim and this can often be achieved simply by maintaining an open airway with jaw thrust or chin lift manoeuvres, and giving oxygen. If ventilatory drive is impaired, bag and mask ventilation may be all that is required.
2. Unskilled attempts at intubation, particularly in the small child, may lead to bruising and oedema of the pharynx and larynx and avoidable hypoxia.
3. The cervical spine must be protected if a neck injury is suspected (see page 256).

Technique

- Nasal intubation should only be done by those skilled in its use and it is usually performed as a secondary procedure (e.g. for transport or longer-term ventilation in the intensive care unit). Nasal intubation provides more stable tube fixation but is more difficult than orotracheal intubation. Consequently only the latter procedure is discussed below.
- Apparatus: make sure all tube connectors, circuits, etc. are compatible. Two functioning laryngoscopes appropriate to the child and a selection of tracheal tubes should be available. In conditions such as croup or epiglottitis, a tube much narrower than predicted is sometimes required. Formulae for calculating the length and diameter of the tube are given in Box 20.3.
- Smaller children are generally intubated using a straight-blade laryngoscope. It has a smaller cross-section and is more readily accommodated in the mouth of an infant. The straight blade allows the large epiglottis of an infant to be lifted to view the vocal cords. The blade is passed into the oesophagus and then gently withdrawn until the larynx drops into view. In larger infants (over 6 months old), the straight blade may be positioned anterior to the epiglottis (in the vallecula) in the same way that the curved-blade laryngoscope is used. The curved blade is usually preferred in children over 2 years old.
- Babies should be intubated with the head in the *neutral* position. Flexion or extension of the neck or atlanto-occipital joint may cause

Box 20.3 *Choice of tracheal tube in children*

TUBE DIAMETER:

$$\text{internal diameter (mm)} = \frac{\text{age (years)}}{4} + 4$$

or the size of the child's little finger

TUBE LENGTH:

$$\text{Length (cm)} = \frac{\text{age (years)}}{2} + 12$$

partial airway obstruction and obscure the view of the airway through the laryngoscope.

- The head should be immobilized with sandbags or by an assistant, otherwise the left hand holding the laryngoscope will be occupied keeping the head still.

Pre-oxygenation is essential

- The laryngoscope is introduced into the mouth, displacing the tongue to the left so that it does not encroach on the view.
- As described above, the tip of the blade is positioned either under the epiglottis (straight blade) or in the vallecula (straight or curved blade), and the larynx is lifted with force applied at 45° towards the junction of the opposite wall and ceiling – leverage would injure the teeth and gums.

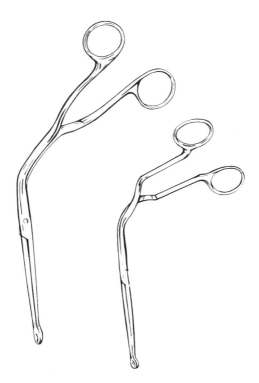

Fig. 20.1 *Magill forceps.*

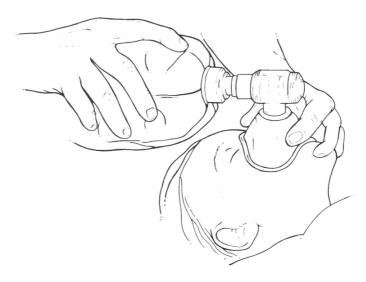

Fig. 20.2 *Bag–valve–mask ventilation for an older child.*

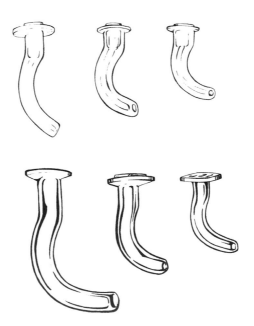

Fig. 20.3 *Oropharyngeal airways: sizes appropriate for children are 000, 00, 0, 1, 1A, 2, 3.*

- The tracheal tube should be introduced gently but firmly.
- If laryngeal spasm is present, intubation may be difficult without traumatizing the larynx: a small diameter tube should be used in these cases.
- Small tubes, particularly those less than 4 mm internal diameter, may need to be stiffened with a plastic-coated aluminium stylet which should not protrude from the end of the tube. Inexperienced staff will find this helpful.
- Once in place, the tracheal tube must be secured with adhesive tape, preferably elasticated. The skin can be protected by applying lighter adhesive tape first.
- Magill forceps (Fig. 20.1) may be used to guide a tracheal tube through the cords or remove a foreign body. The handles should be held at an angle so as not to obscure the view down the airway.

Fears about the complications of prolonged high-flow oxygen therapy are not relevent in the A&E department
A good maxim is that high-flow oxygen should always be the first and last drug

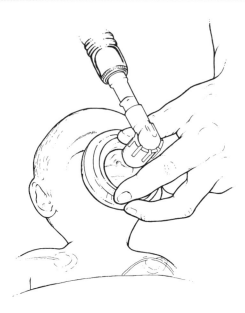

Fig. 20.4   *Bag–valve–mask ventilation in an infant.*

Needle cricothyrotomy

See Practical Procedures, Chapter 28.

Cricothyrotomy insufflation through a cannula is not possible using a self-inflating bag

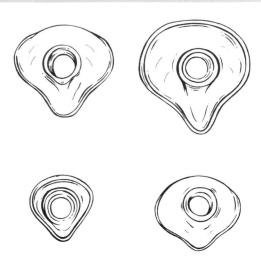

Fig. 20.5 *Masks of various sizes.*

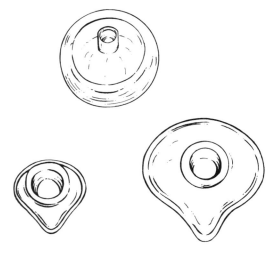

Fig. 20.6 *Ventilation masks.*

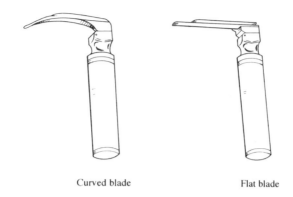

Curved blade   Flat blade

Fig. 20.7 *Laryngoscopes.*

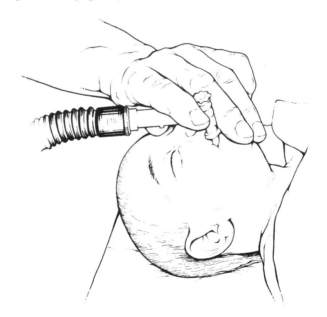

Fig. 20.8 *Ventilation of a child.*

21 CIRCULATORY PROBLEMS

BACKGROUND INFORMATION

- *Shock* is a clinical syndrome resulting form impaired tissue perfusion which is a consequence of acute circulatory failure.
- It may be the end result of many disease processes.
- Impaired delivery of nutrients and oxygen to tissues leads to anaerobic metabolism and acidosis with consequent organ failure and coma unless recognition and intervention are prompt.
- Shock is a progressive syndrome that is artifically divided into three phases:

  1. Compensated shock: vital organ function is conserved by *sympathetic reflexes* which increase systemic arterial resistance and heart rate to maintain cardiac output. Water is preserved through the renin–angiotensin system.
  2. Uncompensated shock: the above mechanisms start to fail and anaerobic metabolism supervenes, resulting in systemic acidosis. Acidosis further reduces myocardial function and impairs the heart's response to catecholamines. Homeostatic mechanisms begin to fail.
  3. Irreversible shock: this is a retrospective diagnosis. Damage to organs is irreversible despite therapeutic intervention.

> Early recognition and effective treatment of shock are vital

The clinical syndrome of shock can develop and progress particularly rapidly in children for two reasons:

1. Children have approximately 80 ml of blood per kg body weight. The loss of a relatively small amount of blood (or fluid) may comprise a large percentage of intravascular volume.
2. Children initially compensate well for fluid loss. As a result there may be few clinical signs until more than a third of circulatory

volume is lost, when progression through the stages of shock may become rapid.

The most common causes of shock in childhood are hypovolaemia and septicaemia. Important causes are listed in Table 21.1.

Table 21.1 *Important causes of shock*

Cardiogenic	Hypovolaemic	Vessel abnormality	Flow restriction	Inadequate oxygen release
Heart failure	Haemorrhage	Septicaemia	Tension	Severe anaemia
Valve disease	Gastroenteritis	Anaphylaxis	pneumothorax	Carbon
Cardiomyopathy	Diabetes	Drugs (e.g.	Pulmonary	monoxide
Arrythmias	Burns	barbiturates)	embolism	poisoning
		Spinal cord	Hypertension	Methaemo-
		injury	Cardiac	globinaemia
			tamponade	

RESUSCITATION

The initial management of the shocked child follows the same pattern irrespective of the precise cause. The history can be established during resuscitation following the ususal 'ABC' approach (Chapter 19 outlines the ABC approach to resuscitation and Chapter 20 covers airway and breathing problems).

Seek help from senior staff

The flow diagram in Fig. 21.1 outlines the initial approach to resuscitation and diagnostic assessment of the shocked child.

DIAGNOSTIC APPROACH

See Fig. 21.1

Investigations

Investigations take second place to assessment and resuscitation.

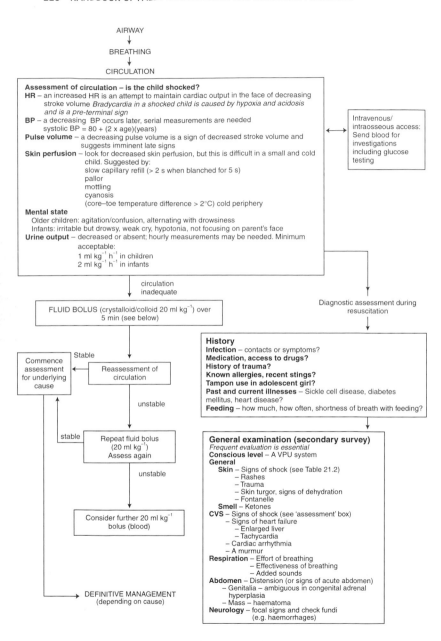

Fig. 21.1 *General management of shock. (BP, blood pressure; CVS, cardiovascular system; HR, heart rate)*

Blood tests

- **Glucose**: The stress of shock often leads to hyperglycaemia. Hypoglycaemia may mimic and coexist with hypovolaemia and may occur in diabetes or Reye's syndrome.
- **Full blood count and differential white cell count**: the haemoglobin level is usually normal in acute blood loss but the packed cell volume is raised when there is fluid loss. The white cell count is often raised (but may be low) in severe sepsis. Disseminated intravascular coagulation (DIC) may cause thrombocytopenia.
- **U&E, creatinine**: electrolyte disturbance depends upon aetiology. Dehydration may induce various alterations in the electrolyte levels.
- **Calcium, phosphate**: hypocalcaemia is common in shock and compromises myocardial and respiratory function.
- **Clotting studies**: hypoxia and acidosis tend to prolong prothrombin and activated partial thromboplastin times, cause DIC and raise levels of fibrinogen degradation products.
- **Blood cultures** may confirm septicaemia.
- **Arterial blood gas analysis**: greater acidosis indicates more severe tissue hypoperfusion.
- **Blood crossmatch/group and save**.
- Others:
    ammonia should be requested in cases of encephalopathy as a marker for Reye's syndrome
    amylase levels may be raised in the occasional case of childhood pancreatitis
    liver function tests may be abnormal in Reye's syndrome

Other investigations

- **Urine culture** (ideally a suprapubic sample).
- A **stool culture** may be considered.
- Appropriate **swabs** (e.g. vaginal if toxic shock syndrome suspected).
- **Lumbar puncture** may be needed, but should be delayed in a shocked patient.
- **Chest X-ray** is likely to show pulmonary plethora (increased lung marking) in cardiac shock, consolidation in pneumonia or abnormal heart shape in congenital heart disease.

- An **ECG** may indicate abnormality of rhythms (e.g. supraventricular tachycardia).

Monitoring

The following should be monitored:

- **Glasgow coma score.**
- Routine nursing and other observations – **pulse, blood pressure, capillary refill time, heart rate, respiratory rate.**
- **Electrocardiogram.**
- **Pulse oximetry.**
- **Central venous pressure** – where there is poor response to fluid therapy or established shock (by experienced personnel only and after resuscitation procedures established).
- **Urine output.**

MANAGEMENT AND REFERRAL

Further management is dependent upon the identified cause (Box 21.1) but the aim is to improve circulatory status by:

1. Increasing circulatory volume (hypovolaemia is the commonest cause of shock in children).
2. Use of drugs to increase cardiac contractility.
3. Removal of outflow obstruction (e.g. pneumothorax).
4. Improving oxygen-carrying capacity.

Methods of managing shock depend on the cause. The following major clinical situations are discussed in this chapter.

1. Hypovolaemic shock
2. Septic shock
3. Anaphylactic shock
4. Cardiogenic shock
5. Diabetic ketoacidosis

See Chapter 7 for the management of gastroenteritis and Chapter 18 for the management of burns

OUTCOME AND PROGNOSIS

Outcome is dependent upon the underlying cause but there is no doubt prompt recognition and treatment of shock will improve prognosis.

HYPOVOLAEMIC SHOCK

BACKGROUND INFORMATION

- Hypovolaemic shock is the commonest cause of shock in infancy and childhood.
- It is due to loss of circulatory volume from any cause.
- It may be due to loss of blood (internal/external haemorrhage), plasma (burns) or dehydration from gastroenteritis, peritonitis, diabetes mellitus or diabetes insipidus.
- Never automatically attribute hypovolaemic shock to isolated head injury.

DIAGNOSTIC APPROACH

A guide to the assessment of signs is given in Table 21.2.

Table 21.2 *Assessment of signs*

	Blood volume deficit		
	10–25%	25–40%	> 40%
Skin	Cool, pale, no sweat	Cold, mottled, mild sweat	Cold, very pale, ashen
Urine output	1 ml kg^{-1} h^{-1}	1 ml kg^{-1} h^{-1}	Possibly nil
Pulse	Slightly weak, tachycardia	Tachycardia, decreased volume	Thready or absent, tachycardia or bradycardia
Systolic BP	Normal	Normal, ?falling	Hypotension
Capillary refill time	2–3 s	4–5 s	> 6 s
Respiratory rate	Mildly tachypnoeic	Tachypnoeic	Sighing respiration
CNS	Lethargic, may show mild agitation	Lethargic, unco-operative	Reacts only to pain, ?comatose

MANAGEMENT

- Initial assessment and resuscitation as indicated above (beware hypoglycaemia which may mimic or coexist with hypovolaemia).
- Use warmed fluids whenever possible.
- Consider transfusion (if appropriate).
- Consider ventilation if no response after two boluses of fluid; CVP monitoring may be required.
- Correct acidosis if pH below 7.15 (use bicarbonate according to the formula in Box 21.1 on p. 239).
- Consider the need for surgery.

SEPTIC SHOCK

BACKGROUND INFORMATION

- Cardiac output may be normal or raised, but still too small to deliver oxygen effectively because of abnormal distribution of blood.

- Causes: Gram-negative bacteria are most frequently responsible but Gram-positive organisms occasionally occur, e.g. haemolytic streptococci, staphylococci. *Neisseria meningitidis* and *Haemophilus influenzae* (incidence declining) are the two most common bacterial causes of septic shock in previously well children.

DIAGNOSTIC APPROACH

The differential diagnosis includes:
- cardiac problems (dysrhythmias)
- congenital heart disease (cardiomyopathy)
- metabolic disorders (hypoglycaemia, electrolyte disturbance e.g. congenital adrenal hyperplasia)
- gastrointestinal problems (volvulus, intussusception)
- severe child abuse
- severe anaemia (haemolytic uraemic syndrome)
- Reye's syndrome
- haemorrhagic shock encephalopathy syndrome.

MANAGEMENT

- Adequate fluid, especially colloids, should be given early in treatment; 60 ml kg^{-1} may be needed.
- Give oxygen 100% via face-mask; consider ventilation.
- Broad-spectrum antibiotic cover is needed (Table 21.3). A broad-spectrum cephalosporin antibiotic (such as cefotaxime or ceftriaxone) is appropriate 'blind' treatment in most cases.
- Inotropic agents can be considered, but only when 60 ml kg^{-1} of fluid has been administered, and not usually in the A&E department.
- Monitor glucose, calcium, bicarbonate and blood gases and treat as appropriate.

Table 21.3 *Guidelines for antibiotic therapy*

Age (months)	Antibiotics
< 1	Cefotaxime (100 mg kg^{-1} $dose^{-1}$)
	Some consider ampicillin and gentamicin in this age group because of the wider range of more unusual organisms in the neonatal period
	Advice should be sought from senior A&E; paediatric or microbiological staff
1–3	Cefotaxime or ceftriaxone (25–50 mg kg^{-1} $dose^{-1}$)
	Some consider ampicillin also in this age group to cover organisms such as *Listeria*
> 3	Cefotaxime or ceftriaxone (25–50 mg kg^{-1} $dose^{-1}$)
	Benzylpenicillin (50 mg kg^{-1}) if meningococcal septicaemia suspected

ANAPHYLACTIC SHOCK

BACKGROUND INFORMATION

Anaphylactic shock is immunologically mediated and commonly caused by allergy to drugs (pencillin in particular), contrast media and foods (especially nuts).

DIAGNOSTIC APPROACH

Symptoms may begin with itching (lips, mouth) and nausea, associated with an urticarial rash or angio-oedema, and progress through sweating, irritability, wheezing, and loose motions to collapse. The signs are those of shock (pallor, tachycardia) and of bronchospasm/laryngeal oedema.

MANAGEMENT

The management principles follow the same initial assessment as outlined above (oxygen and assessment of 'ABC').

1. Remove allergen.
2. Assess 'ABC' – address airway and breathing problems as identified; consider intubation or surgical airway, particularly if stridor is marked.
3. Give adrenaline 10 µg kg^{-1} im followed by 5 ml 1:1000 nebulized adrenaline.
4. Give nebulized salbutamol 5 mg at once (repeated every 15 min while wheezy).
5. Give colloid 20 ml kg^{-1} if clinical evidence of shock.
6. Reassess 'ABC' and consider repeat adrenaline 10 µg kg^{-1} if child is still wheezy; give the dose intravenously if intravenous access secured and shock is life-threatening, or previous im dose ineffective.
7. If child is still wheezy give hydrocortisone 4 mg kg^{-1} iv and consider infusion, aminophylline or salbutamol or adrenaline.

CARDIOGENIC SHOCK

BACKGROUND INFORMATION

- Cardiogenic shock results when the heart fails to deliver sufficient nutrients to the body as a result of primary cardiac dysfunction.
- The commonest causes in childhood are:
  dysrhythmias (e.g. supraventricular tachycardia)
  congenital heart disease that obstructs the left ventricular outflow tract (e.g. coarctation of the aorta)
  damage to the myocardium from poisons (e.g. tricyclic antidepressants)
  following cardiopulmonary resuscitation (due to hypoxia/ischaemia)
  as a result of myocarditis or cardiomyopathy
  following septic shock (possibly due to release of toxins)

DIAGNOSTIC APPROACH

In addition to the features already mentioned, the following features may be present and should be sought in any child with a suggestive history:

hepatomegaly
gallop rhythm
pulmonary oedema
jugular venous distension

These features are all suggestive of circulatory overload (pump failure).

MANAGEMENT AND REFERRAL

The management should be under the guidance of senior A&E and paediatric staff and the child should be transferred to the intensive care unit as soon as initial resuscitation procedures have ensured stabilization. The *principles* of treatment only are outlined below.

- Improve oxygen supply to the heart:
  give 100% oxygen via face-mask; consider early intubation and mechanical ventilation to reduce excessive work of breathing (and reduce oxygen requirement)
  transfuse anaemic patients (packed cells)
  reduce oxygen requirement (e.g. relief of pain)
- Correct abnormalities of electrolytes, blood glucose and arterial blood gases (acidosis).
- Treat hypotension with plasma 10 ml kg^{-1} and repeat as necessary (CVP monitoring may be required); maintain urine output (at least 1 ml kg^{-1} h^{-1} with fluids, diuretics and dopamine infusions).
- Support myocardial function with inotropes (e.g. dopamine with or without dobutamine, adrenaline, isoprenaline).
- Reduce afterload with sedation and vasodilators (e.g. nitro-prusside).

DIABETIC KETOACIDOSIS

BACKGROUND INFORMATION

- Ketoacidosis is found at presentation in approximately 30% of newly diagnosed diabetic children and may occur in known diabetic patients as a result of illness, infection or poor management of the disease.
- Hyperglycaemia and osmotic diuresis are caused by an absolute or relative lack of insulin and cause severe dehydration. The child may present in a severly shocked state.
- In addition, in the absence of insulin, fat metabolism results in the production of large quantities of ketones and metabolic acidosis. Initially, the latter is compensated for by hyperventilation and respiratory alkalosis until the compensatory mechanisms cannot cope and coma supervenes.

RESUSCITATION

- The initial assessment should follow the general guidelines outlined above.
- The diagnosis will be suspected in any shocked (dehydrated) child with a high blood glucose concentration during testing in the initial stages of resuscitation.
- It is normal to use 4.5% albumin as the resuscitation fluid (for restoration of circulatory volume) in cases of suspected diabetic ketoacidosis (DKA).

> The priority of management is correction of shock
> Definitive management of fluids and insulin should not be
> commenced until shock is corrected

DIAGNOSTIC APPROACH

The typical presentation will have the following features:

- A history of **polydipsia**, **polyuria** and **recent weight loss** may be obtained.
- **Abdominal pain** and **vomiting** may be present (it may be mis-diagnosed as an 'acute abdomen').
- A **rapid respiratory rate** (sometimes mistaken for pneumonia or asthma) or **Kussmaul respiration** (deep, rapid breathing).

Clinical assessment should be directed towards assessing the **degree of shock/dehydration**, **neurological assessment** (coma scale) and **identification of a possible focus of infection** after initial resuscitation procedures.

Initial investigations should include:

> **blood glucose** test
> **U&E/bicarbonate**
> **arterial blood gases**
> **full blood count, packed cell volume**
> **urinalysis** and **culture**

A **full septic screen** may be required in a pyrexial child.

Careful monitoring is required as described above, particularly:

> strict **fluid balance** measurements
> hourly **blood glucose** measurements
> half-hourly **neurological observations**
> **ECG monitoring** (T wave changes accompany dangerous hypokalaemia)

MANAGEMENT AND REFERRAL

After correction of shock the following management problems need to be considered.

Fluid management

Calculate the amount of fluid needed as the maintenance requirements plus the fluid deficit, which is estimated according to the formula in Box 21.1. Maintenance fluids can be estimated from weight using the table on p. 364.

- Ignore any fluids given during the initial resuscitation.
- Overzealous fluid replacement is a risk factor for cerebral oedema, so calculate the deficit as if the patient is no more than 10% dehydrated.
- The type of fluid used should be 0.9% saline until the blood glucose level has fallen to 12 mmol l^{-1}, at this point change to 0.45% saline with 5% dextrose.
- Catheterization is unecessary unless there is evidence of a palpable bladder, a comatose patient, or no urine output 4 hours after commencing treatment.

Correction of acidosis

Continuing acidosis is an indication of inadequate resuscitation and bicarbonate correction should be rarely needed. It may be considered for a profoundly acidotic child (pH < 6.9), in which case a half-correction of the acidosis should be made (using 8.4% sodium bicarbonate over 60 min) according to the formula in Box 21.1. Check with senior staff if this management option is considered.

Box 21.1 *Volume calculations for fluid management and correction of acidosis*

FLUID DEFICIT

Deficit (ml) = dehydration (%) × body weight (kg) × 10
  (i.e. 10 kg infant 7.5% dehydrated needs 750 ml replacement)

Ignore amount of fluids given during initial resuscitation

Give 0.9% saline when blood glucose concentration > 12 mmol l^{-1}

Give 0.45% saline plus 5% dextrose when blood glucose
  ⩽ 12 mmol l^{-1}

CORRECTION OF ACIDOSIS

Volume of bicarbonate (ml) =

$$\frac{\frac{1}{3} \text{body weight (kg)} \times \text{base deficit (mmol l}^{-1})}{2}$$

Give as 8.4% sodium bicarbonate over 60 min

Potassium replacement

Potassium replacement should commence immediately (20 mmol KCl to every 500 ml bag of fluid) unless anuria is suspected. Cardiac monitoring is mandatory (for T wave changes) and plasma electrolytes should be checked every 2 h.

Insulin

Fluid replacement is the priority in the A&E department and the paediatric staff should usually have taken over care at this stage. Once the blood glucose result is known it is usual to infuse insulin at a rate of 0.1 unit kg^{-1} h^{-1} (50 ml human soluble insulin, e.g. Actrapid, added to 50 ml 0.9% saline in a syringe pump and infused at a rate of 0.1 ml kg^{-1} h^{-1}). The rate should be reduced to 0.05 units kg^{-1} h^{-1} if the rate of fall of the blood glucose exceeds 5 mmol h^{-1} or when the blood glucose level drops to 12 mmol l^{-1}. If the blood glucose level falls to 7 mmol l^{-1} or below the insulin should not be stopped but extra glucose should be added to the infusion fluid.

Cerebral oedema

Clinical features of cerebral oedema include:

> headache
> confusion
> irritability
> reduced conscious level
> small pupils
> slowing pulse (but rising blood pressure)
> papilloedema

Refer managment to senior staff as fluid management may need to be adjusted (to two-thirds of maintenance levels once shock has been treated), mannitol may be required (0.5 g kg^{-1} every 6 h, given as 2.5 ml kg^{-1} 20% of mannitol over 15 min), other diagnoses may need to be excluded (e.g. by CT scan) and intensive care management will be required.

Antibiotics

Antibiotics may be required if there is evidence of infection, preferably after obtaining as much of a septic screen as possible, but omitting a lumbar puncture if there is evidence of depressed consciousness.

OUTCOME AND PROGNOSIS

In general, the earlier effective intervention is achieved, the better the outcome from diabetic ketoacidosis.

22 IMPAIRED CONSCIOUSNESS

BACKGROUND INFORMATION

- The term 'altered mental state' refers to an alteration in a patient's level of consciousness and always implies serious pathology.
- Terms such as 'delirium', 'stupor', 'obtunded' and 'drowsy' are often loosely applied (and defined) and so scoring systems have been developed to determine the degree of altered mental state more precisely. The most widely used systems are the Glasgow coma scale and the modified children's coma scale (see Chapter 14 and Part VI).
- These scales are semiquantitive and are difficult to apply rapidly in the urgent situations encountered in the A&E department. Determination of conscious level in these instances needs to be kept as simple as possible and should enable the child to be placed into one of the four 'AVPU' categories:

> **A**LERT
> Responds to **V**OICE
> Responds to **P**AIN
> **U**NRESPONSIVE

- Ninety-five per cent of patients in coma have usually suffered a diffuse injury to the brain. The causes are shown in Box 22.1
- Structural lesions account for only 5% of cases.

RESUSCITATION

- The initial assessment of the child with altered mental state follows the standard pattern, the principles being maintenance of Airway, Breathing and Circulation (see Chapter 19) and prevention of secondary brain damage, e.g. raised intracranial pressure.

> Seek help early from senior A&E or paediatric staff

Box 22.1 *Causes of coma*

COMMON CAUSES

NEUROLOGICAL: epilepsy, head injury (accidental/non-accidental)

INFECTIVE: meningoencephalitis, septicaemia, gastroenteritis

METABOLIC: poisoning (drugs, alcohol, glue, etc.)

UNCOMMON CAUSES

NEUROLOGICAL: brain abscess, vascular accidents, tumour, hydrocephalus

METABOLIC: Electrolyte disturbance, inborn errors of metabolism, thyroid/adrenal disorders, Reye's syndrome

OTHERS: hypoxia/hypercapnia, intussusception, hypothermia, hypertension, hysteria

- The principles of resuscitation are as outlined in the preceding chapters:

1. AIRWAY – an adequate airway must be maintained (see Chapter 20).

> Cervical spine protection is mandatory in any child obtunded by head injury (see Chapter 23)

2. BREATHING – give high-flow oxygen. Intubate and ventilate if there is no gag reflex, if the Glasgow coma scale score is less than 8 or breathing is inadequate (see Chapter 20).
3. CIRCULATION – establish iv access (and collect blood samples). Treat shock as in Chapter 21 with 20 ml kg^{-1} of fluid.

Initial blood investigations are FBC, clotting, U&E, calcium, glucose, blood culture, group and save.

> Treatment of shock is the priority but in its absence, fluid should be restricted (2 ml kg^{-1} h^{-1} or about $\frac{2}{3}$ of normal maintenance fluids)

- **Hypoglycaemia** is the next priority: a glucose level below 4 mmol l^{-1} is treated with 5 ml kg^{-1} of 10% glucose (after taking a sample for laboratory analysis). In older children 2 ml kg^{-1} of 25% glucose can be used. Beware potential osmotic effects of high concentrations.
- Rapid neurological assessment:
  if **unresponsive**, consider immediate intubation and ventilation, a rapid and brief **history** and **examination** are required: look for readily identifiable and treatable causes (e.g. trauma to the head, purpuric rash of meningococcal septicaemia, a history of diabetes or epilepsy, or a possible history of poisoning)
- Reassessment of 'ABC' and a **fuller rapid neurological assessment** should take place at this stage:
  Glasgow coma scale or children's coma scale
  pupil responses
  posture

> The important issues during the primary survey are maintenance of ABC and 'treating the treatable'

- After the primary survey a fuller diagnostic assessment (secondary survey) should be made.

DIAGNOSTIC APPROACH

If the situation is stable a **secondary survey** takes place, which involves a more detailed history, examination and investigation to establish the cause of the coma.

> Regular re-evaluation of ABC and neurological status must take place during the secondary survey

The primary survey must be repeated if there is any change in the patient's condition.

History

Focus on identifying the underlying abnormality. The following are important:

- **History of the current illness or injury**:
  infectious contact
  recent trauma and/or head injury (see Chapter 14).
  recent general health: history of fever
  health prior to the precipitating event
  associated symptoms: vomiting, diarrhoea, respiratory difficulty
- **Previous medical history**:
  known previous illness: diabetes, epilepsy, renal disease, heart
      disease
  similar episodes in the past (e.g. previous prolonged febrile fit)?
  could there be an underlying inborn error of metabolism?
  history of depressive illness or eating disorder
  travel abroad
  regular medication (e.g. antiepileptic drugs)?

Examination

- **Basic observations** must be recorded followed by a **general examination** as in Part I. Specific examination focuses on assessing neurological impairment and identifying the cause.
- Examination should be systematic and a 'head to toe' approach is recommended:

Head

- Observe and palpate for **wound**, **haematoma** or **fracture**.
- Palpate the anterior fontanelle in an infant for **fullness**, **depression** or **pulsation** (which may give an indication of dehydration or raised intracranial pressure).

Eyes

- Look at **eye position**:
      in cerebral lesions eyes deviate towards a destructive lesion and
      away from an irritative lesion

in brain stem lesions eyes deviate away from a destructive lesion

- Look at **pupil reaction**:

  fixed dilated pupils – hypoxia, hypotension, hypothermia, cerebral oedema, midbrain lesion, post-seizure anticholinergic drugs

  pinpoint pupils – opioid or organophosphate poisoning, metabolic disorders, pontine damage

  unilateral fixed dilated pupils – epilepsy and mass lesions such as subdural, tentorial herniation

- Look at **fundi**:

  normal fundi do not exclude raised intracranial pressure

  look for **haemorrhage** and **papilloedema**

- Look at **reflex ocular movements**:

  in patients without head or neck injury the **oculocephalic reflexes** should be assessed; abnormality may indicate raised intracranial pressure

  in normal individuals, rotation or flexion of head left or right should result in movement of eyes *away* from direction of movement

Ears, nose

Look for evidence of **bleeding** to indicate basal fracture.

Neck

Examine for **swelling**, **bruising**, **deformity** and, in the absence of trauma, **rigidity** (which might suggest meningeal irritation). Auscultate for **bruits** in the neck.

Skin

- Examine for **petechiae** or **purpura** which might suggest meningo-coccal septicaemia.
- Examine for **jaundice** or **signs of trauma**.
- Occasionally an **odour** may reveal a metabolic disorder or poisoning.

Chest

- Examine for signs of **respiratory illness** (see Chapter 6).
- **Hyperventilation** occurs as a compensation in metabolic acidosis (e.g. diabetic ketoacidosis or severe salicylate toxicity).
- **Cheyne–Stokes** respiration signifies bilateral hemisphere abnormality with intact brain stem. This may herald respiratory arrest.

Abdomen

Examine for **hepatosplenomegaly**, **abdominal mass**, **distension**, **rigidity**, reduced **bowel sounds**.

Neurological examination

- Examination of **eyes** (see above).
- Examination of **posture** may suggest the location of the lesion:
  asymmetry of movement should be noted
       dysfunction of cerebral hemisphere may cause arms to be **flexed** and legs **extended**
       extension of both upper and lower extremities implies decorticate posturing
- **Tone** may be **increased** and **reflexes** may be exaggerated in raised intracranial pressure, with **up-going toes** (i.e. abnormal plantar reflexes).
- **Tone** may be **decreased**, with **down-going toes** (i.e. a normal plantar reflex) if metabolic causes or drugs.

Investigations

- **Blood samples**: FBC, glucose, U&E, calcium/magnesium, blood cultures, arterial blood gases, liver enzymes, blood ammonia, paracetamol and salicylate levels, blood alcohol.
- **Urine samples**: cultures (MC&S), metabolic screen (for organic and amino acids), toxicology.
- **Radiography**: CXR (plus other X-rays if history of trauma), CT brain scan (possibly).
- **Continued monitoring**: basic observations (pulse, blood pressure, ECG, respiratory rate), pluse oximetry, fluid balance, coma score.

Note: lumbar puncture is *contraindicated* until raised intracranial pressure is excluded.

MANAGEMENT AND REFERRAL

Senior help should be sought at all stages of management

The priority is to treat identifiable causes. This should involve treatment with **broad-spectrum intravenous antibiotics** (e.g. cefotaxime or ceftriaxone) in all cases where sepsis is a possibility.

Whatever the cause of coma, it is vital to maintain homeostasis:

maintain good oxygenation and circulation
normalize acid base and electrolyte balance
maintain blood glucose
maintain body temperature
detect and treat raised intracranial pressure (see below)

Raised intracranial pressure

Raised intracranial pressure (ICP) is a common accompaniment of most causes of coma, due to cerebral oedema or an expanding space-occupying lesion (e.g. haematoma).

- The aims of treatment are to maintain adequate cerebral blood flow. This is dependent upon cerebral perfusion pressure (mean arterial pressure minus intracranial pressure) and cerebrovascular resistance (in turn, often impaired by trauma, hypoxia or ischaemia).
- Methods of management – obtain specialist advice about the following:
    nursing 'head up' (30°)
    consider mild hyperventilation to maintain low to normal level of $P\text{CO}_2$
    mannitol 0.25–0.5 g kg^{-1} (50% 0.5 ml kg^{-1} in 30 min)

sedation and pain relief to prevent surges in ICP
dexamethasone 400 µg kg^{-1} every 6 h may be helpful

OUTCOME AND PROGNOSIS

Outcome and prognosis depend upon the cause (some of which are discussed below), but there is no doubt prompt intervention will improve
the prognosis.

MENINGITIS AND ENCEPHALITIS

BACKGROUND INFORMATION

- Eighty per cent of all bacterial meningitis occurs in childhood.
  Children also develop viral meningitis.
- Encephalitis is usually viral or secondary to other infections and is
  characterized by fever, disturbed consciousness, convulsions and
  focal neurological signs.
- Many of the signs and symptoms of severe meningitis are primarily
  those of raised intracranial pressure.
- Problems to consider:
    1. Seizures.
    2. Inappropriate antidiuretic hormone (ADH) secretion and elec-
        trolyte imbalance.
    3. Septicaemic shock.
    4. Subdural effusions.
    5. Cerebral oedema.
    6. Neurological sequelae.
    7. Prophylaxis for contacts.

Causes

Causes may be acute bacterial (Box 22.2) viral (echo-, mumps, coxsackieviruses), tuberculosis or fungal.

Box 22.2 *Causes of bacterial meningitis by age*

NEONATAL (< 1 MONTH)

E. coli, Gram–negative organisms

Group B streptococci

Listeria monocytogenes

OVER 3 MONTHS

Neisseria meningitidis

Streptococcus pneumoniae

Haemophilus influenzae (usually < 6 years – less common now with HiB vaccine)

1–3 MONTHS

Any of the above

DIAGNOSTIC APPROACH

Neonate, infant

Symptoms are non-specific: fever, poor feeding, irritability, vomiting, full fontanelle, drowsiness, apnoea, convulsions, rash.

Older child

Classical signs may be present: headache, vomiting, neck stiffness, photophobia, coma, convulsions, rash, fever.

MANAGEMENT AND REFERRAL

- Full septic screen (see Chapter 5) is needed, ideally prior to antibiotics – but the priority is antibiotic treatment. Do not forget to obtain a throat swab and remember that lumbar puncture should be deferred if raised intracranial pressure cannot be excluded.

- A broad-spectrum antibiotic should be given (usually cefotaxime or ceftriaxone in the A&E department). Some paediatricians advocate ampicillin when *Listeria* is suspected and antibiotic treatment can be reviewed at a later stage.
- Transfer to specialist care should be in the company of suitably skilled staff and the disease needs to be notified to the Public Health Laboratory (PHL). Close contacts will need to be treated with antibiotic prophylaxis (usually rifampicin) as directed by a microbiologist.

STATUS EPILEPTICUS

BACKGROUND INFORMATION

- Status epilepticus is defined as a single convulsion lasting longer than 30 min or a series of convulsions (of similar duration) during which the patient does not fully regain consciousness.
- It is more common in childhood than adulthood. Up to 5% of children under 15 years old with epilepsy will have an episode of status epilepticus and up to 10% of children having febrile fits present in status epilepticus.
- The majority of cases occur under the age of 2 years and often this is the first seizure.
- Causes include:

    1. Febrile convulsions.
    2. 'Acute' brain dysfunction (e.g. CNS infection, encephalopathies, metabolic/toxic causes, trauma, cerebrovascular accident, electrolyte disorders).
    3. 'Chronic' CNS disorders (e.g. cerebral palsy, tumour).
    4. Other causes (e.g. sudden decrease in antiepileptic medication or excess administration of local anaesthetic).

    As a rough guide, each of the above four groups of causes accounts for roughly a quarter of all cases.

- The incidence of serious sequelae is primarily related to the under-lying cause, the majority of complications occurring in the group with 'acute' brain dysfunction. The incidence of complications is also higher in those under 6 months old.
- Overall approximately two-thirds of children with status epilepticus lasting more than 60 min will have irreversible neurological handicap. Thus the principle of management is to stop the fit before that time and preferably before 45 min have expired.

DIAGNOSTIC APPROACH

- The diagnosis of status epilepticus is made on the definition above. Note that the fits can be grand mal, partial or focal.
- The approach to diagnosing the underlying cause should follow the principles outlined in Chapters 2 and 3.
- A careful history from accompanying adults and a thorough head to toe examination are essential.

Investigations

- The following investigations are *recommended*: **FBC**, **U&E** (including bicarbonate), measurements of **glucose**, **magnesium**, **calcium** and **phosphate**. Electrolyte disturbances, hypoglycaemia or a raised white cell count may be revealed.
- *Consider*:

> **septic screen** (see Chapter 5), particularly in a pyrexial child
> a **metabolic screen**
> **liver function tests/ammonia levels** (to exclude Reye's syndrome)
> **clotting studies**
> **toxicology** (urine or blood)
> **CT scan** of the brain
> **anticonvulsant levels** may also be appropriate

- Monitoring: **blood pressure**, **temperature** (core temperature if possible), **pulse oximetry** (plus possibly arterial blood gas analysis), **ECG** and **urine output**.

MANAGEMENT AND REFERRAL

> **MANAGEMENT OF STATUS EPILEPTICUS**
> 1. Maintain 'ABC' while stopping the fit
> 2. Determine the cause
> 3. Treat the cause where possible

The following managment sequence is recommended.

1. Assess ABC (see Chapter 19), while giving a first dose of **rectal diazepam** (0.4 mg kg^{-1}); give high-flow oxygen by face-mask and ventilate if necessary. Rectal diazepam works in approximately 5 min and its effect can last approximately 1 h.

2. Establish **intravenous access** and take a blood sample to send for the tests indicated above; check an immediate **blood glucose level** – if it is below 3 mmol l^{-1} glucose should be given (2 ml kg^{-1} of 25% solution, or 5 ml kg^{-1} of 10% solution). Initiate treatment for shock (if present).

3. Reassess ABC and make a quick assessment of **neurological status** using the AVPU system.

4. In the absence of shock establish an **isotonic fluid infusion** (e.g. dextrose saline) at no more than two-thirds of maintenance rate in order to minimize the risk of cerebral oedema (2 ml kg^{-1} h^{-1} may be appropriate).

5. Repeat the dose of **rectal diazepam** if fitting persists 5 min after the first dose and call for senior help. If iv access has been established the same dose can be given as an iv bolus over 30 s.

6. If fitting persists after a further 5 min a dose of **rectal paraldehyde** (0.2–0.4 ml kg^{-1} as a 50:50 solution in arachis oil) should be given (paraldehyde can also be given intramuscularly but is not recommended as it can cause severe abscess formation).

7. If fitting persists after a further 10 min another anticonvulsant should be given. **Phenytoin** (10–20 mg kg^{-1} iv given over 20–30 min no faster than 1 mg kg^{-1} min^{-1}) is the usual choice – the infusion should be made up with 0.9% saline to a maximum concentration of 1 mg in 1 ml. Phenytoin has a peak action in 1h but a long half-life that is dose-dependent; levels should be measured

90–120 min after completion and blood pressure and ECG monitoring are essential. Care is needed if the patient has been taking oral phenytoin – commence the infusion only if blood levels are less than 2.5 mg ml^{-1}. **Phenobarbitone** (15 mg kg^{-1} iv) is often the preferred choice in neonates but this may also cause a drop in blood pressure.

8. If the patient is still fitting after 30 min of phenytoin infusion (or after a total of 45 min) prepare to paralyse and ventilate (i.e. call the anaesthetist early). A **thiopentone** infusion is appropriate, the loading dose being 4–8 mg kg^{-1} administered by an anaesthetist.

Note: mannitol should be considered by slow iv infusion to decrease intracranial pressure.

- In most cases the patient should receive a loading dose of phenytoin, even if the seizure stops with doses of diazepam.
- In non-convulsive status epilepticus (e.g. continuous complex partial seizures) patients are often resistant to benzodiazepines, but the same sequence should be tried.
- In approximately 80% of cases the fitting will stop after a single dose of diazepam and over 90% of cases can be managed outside ITU using diazepam, paraldehyde and phenytoin.
- Many other drugs may be considered (e.g. clonazepam infusion, lignocaine infusion, chlormethiazole infusion), but the decision to use these rests with senior paediatric staff.

The patient should never be transferred while still fitting

Summary

The usual drug sequence is:

1. Diazepam (pr/iv).
2. Diazepam (pr/iv).
3. Paraldehyde (pr).
4. Phenytoin (or phenobarbitone in neonates) (iv).
5. Anaesthetic (thiopentone).

23 MAJOR TRAUMA

BACKGROUND INFORMATION

- Trauma is a cause of disease that kills more children (over the age of 1 year) than any other.
- Nearly 50% of all trauma deaths occur immediately or within the first few minutes of the accident. Survivors may die within a few hours from potentially remediable conditions involving airway, respiratory and circulatory (ABC) disorders (i.e. hypoxia or shock), raised intracranial pressure or spinal cord damage from failure to immobilize the spine.
- Deaths after days or weeks result from multiple organ failure, fat embolism, pulmonary embolism or sepsis. Good care in the first few hours can help to reduce the number of late deaths.
- Standardized treatment protocols help to provide a structured, logical and co-ordinated approach under stress. A smooth and uninterrupted chain of care from the accident to surgery or intensive care is vital. Prompt resuscitation, investigation and surgical intervention reduce mortality and morbidity.
- A trauma team should be available led by a senior doctor experienced in and committed to trauma care, supported by appropriately trained doctors from relevant specialties (particularly anaesthesia, general surgery, orthopaedic surgery and paediatrics). Senior A&E nurses, radiographers and pathology technicians are also required. The staff should be trained in advanced trauma and paediatric life support.
- Children represent a small target for the dissipation of mechanical forces. As a result, multiorgan injury is the norm and all systems must be considered at risk.
- Advanced trauma life support consists of four phases: the **primary survey**, **resuscitation**, **secondary survey** and definitive care. Although described separately, they merge into each other.

ADVANCED TRAUMA LIFE SUPPORT PROCEDURE

Preparation

Before the patient arrives (if forewarned), summon the trauma team or individual help as defined in your own hospital. Prepare equipment in the resuscitation room and don protective clothing (visor, apron, gloves) until the casualties have been assessed.

Primary survey and resuscitation

The initial assessment follows the sequence of **airway** (with **cervical spine immobilization**), **breathing**, **circulation**, **disability** and **exposure**. It is essential that action is taken on each life-threatening condition as it is identified.

> The primary survey and resuscitation are performed simultaneously

Airway and cervical spine

The first priority in the unconscious child is to open, clear and maintain the airway.

Spinal injury must be assumed until it is proved otherwise, so immobilization of the cervical spine is established or maintained as the airway is opened. If the child responds to questions when hands are placed on each side of the head, the airway is already safe and breathing and circulation are intact. Put the head and neck into a neutral position, if not already in it, by gentle repositioning. Do not apply traction or axial compression of the spine, nor force the head into the neutral position. If a mechanical block, severe pain or neurological symptoms are encountered, call for senior help.

If there is **grunting**, **stridor**, **choking** or **snoring**, ask an assistant to hold the head and neck in neutral while you are attending to the airway. Perform a chin lift or jaw thrust. *Do not use head tilt* which will extend the injured spine and also obstruct the airway in small children. Use suction to remove secretions or blood.

Insertion of a correctly sized oropharyngeal (Guedel) tube can maintain the airway temporarily in the unconscious child, either alone or in combination with chin lift or jaw thrust. Nasopharyngeal tubes have no place in the airway management of small children in an emergency situation.

You will now need anaesthetic help. Oral intubation may be necessary to secure the airway. Rarely, oral intubation performed by an experienced anaesthetist is unsuccessful, usually because of distorted anatomy. A needle cricothyroidotomy should then be established as an emergency procedure. Surgical cricothyroidotomy is contraindicated in children under 12 years old.

Once the airway is secure in the unconscious or co-operative child, **cervical spine immobilization** is assured by applying a correctly sized semirigid collar, supplemented by sandbags or cushions each side of the head, held in place by broad adhesive tapes across the forehead as well as by the chin-piece of the collar. If the child is active and unco-operative, use the collar alone to avoid a struggle (although this provides less protection). In the event of any difficulty (e.g. a very small child), it is safer (and more comforting) to ask someone to hold the head.

Cervical spine immobilization is not removed until cervical X-rays and the peripheral neurological examination are found to be normal. A child in coma cannot co-operate with the neurological examination so immobilization must continue until consciousness returns and the examination can be completed.

Document any **airway manoeuvres** or **adjuncts** employed, as well as the **technique used to control the cervical spine**.

Breathing

Is the child breathing? Assess by observing the chest, listening and feeling for expired air. If the child is breathing, assess the effort and the child's **colour**, and count the **respiratory rate** – you must be aware of the normal rates in children of different ages.

- If breathing is shallow, slow or absent, **ventilate** as necessary using a self-inflating bag fitted with a reservoir and connected to oxygen at 10 l min^{-1}.
- If the child is breathing adequately, apply an **oxygen** mask with a reservoir bag attached. Oxygen **flow** should be 12 l min^{-1} and the F_{IO_2} will then be at 90–95%.

Is there asymmetrical **chest expansion** with breathing or ventilation (suggesting injury on the affected side), or **bruising**, **deformity**, **paradoxical movement** (**flail segment**), **recession** or **accessory muscle use**? Is there a sucking chest **wound**? Look at the **neck veins**.

Palpate the **trachea** which may be deviated to one side by a tension pneumothorax or a haemothorax on the contralateral side. Feel the chest wall for **bony crepitus** (rib fracture), **surgical emphysema** (with air leakage from the pleural space, bronchi or oesophagus), **flail segment** (which may be subtle) or other chest wall defects.

Percuss both sides of the chest for increased **resonance** (possible pneumothorax) or dullness (haemothorax).

Auscultate for **breath sounds**. Absence can indicate a pneumothorax or haemothorax – both are as common in children as they are in adults, but greater mediastinal displacement and compromise occur in children.

Many of these injuries occur in combination. *Surgical assistance is required*.

Particularly important life-threatening chest injuries to be identified at this stage are:

> tension pneumothorax
> haemothorax
> sucking chest wounds
> pericardial tamponade
> flail segment

If examination of the chest reveals:

- A tense, resonant hemithorax with reduced breath sounds, and sometimes respiratory distress, cyanosis and engorged neck veins: **tension pneumothorax** is the clinical diagnosis. Immediately insert a large-bore cannula into the second intercostal space in the midclavicular line (no time for local anaesthesia). A hiss of air indicates success. A chest drain can then be introduced into the fourth or fifth intercostal space in the anterior axillary line under local anaesthesia using the technique of blunt dissection to the pleural cavity, a finger-sweep to break down any adhesions, and insertion of the drain (without the trocar which is discarded) (see Fig. 23.1).

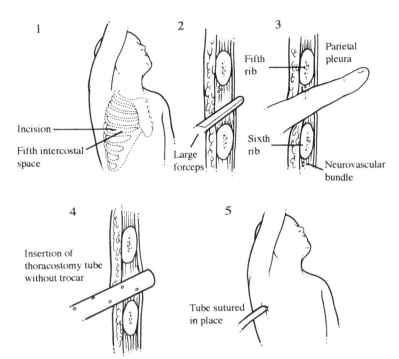

Fig. 23.1

- A dull hemithorax with reduced breath sounds in a shocked child: **haemothorax** is the working diagnosis. Support of the circulation is needed (see below) in addition to chest drain insertion. The source of the bleeding is not important at this stage.
- Visible or palpable paradoxical chest movement: **flail segment** is the diagnosis. This will be accompanied by underlying pulmonary contusion which can develop and progress to cause respiratory failure. The initial chest X-ray is often normal. Blood gases need to be monitored and intensivists are needed to manage the respiratory failure and control pain relief. Bear in mind that ribs are more flexible and fracture less easily in children so pulmonary contusion often develops without any overlying rib fracture.
- Engorged neck veins, tachycardia and a narrowed pulse pressure in a hypotensive child whose heart sounds may be difficult to hear: consider **cardiac tamponade** which is more common in penetrating trauma. Obtain expert help as this is a surgical emergency,

demanding cardiothoracic expertise. Temporary improvement can be gained with pericardiocentesis using a long cannula inserted through the left costoxiphisternal angle with ECG monitoring in place to avoid penetration of the myocardium which can produce arrhythmias. Aspiration of a few millilitres of blood gives temporary respite and a three-way tap allows repeated aspiration.

- A **sucking chest wound**, most commonly from a penetrating injury: this should be covered with an adhesive film dressing such as Opsite or surgical gauze which is not secured on one side. The wound must not be sealed until a chest drain has been inserted, otherwise a tension pneumothorax can develop.

If treating a haemothorax or pneumothorax, insert the first intravenous cannula, take blood samples and start fluids while the **chest drain** is being prepared. The second cannula can be inserted after the chest drain is secure.

Circulation

Deal with 'circulation' only after 'breathing' has been addressed – children die more rapidly from hypoxia than from shock.

- Rapidly assess the **skin**. **Pallor**, **cool or cold skin** and **sweating** are all markers of circulatory **shock**.
- Determine the **capillary refill time**: if longer than 2 s, the peripheral circulation is reduced. Palpate **central and peripheral pulses**. If they are weak, or peripheral pulses are absent, the child is in an advanced stage of shock.

Children with significant blood loss can compensate physiologically and maintain their vital signs within the normal range for a long period. Clinical signs of shock may not appear until the circulating blood volume has decreased by approximately 25%. **Tachycardia** and increased capillary refill times are the earliest pointers to a diagnosis of shock (see Chapter 21) but the former is not always helpful in a stressed child.

Gain **vascular access** immediately. Two large-bore cannulae, the **size** depending on the age of the child, should be inserted into the most prominent veins available. Without delay, take blood from the first cannula for a **full blood count**, **emergency crossmatch**, and estimates of

urea, **electrolytes** and **glucose**. Assessment of the circulation determines the **type of crossmatch** and the **quantity of blood required**.

Start **fluid therapy** directly after blood has been taken. Crystalloids, at a **rate** of 20 ml kg^{-1}, are recommended initially. The fluids should be warmed to body temperature (a warm cabinet or fluid warmer should be available).

If venous access is unsuccessful, **intraosseous needle** insertion in children is a recommended alternative (Chapter 28), and is preferable to a venous cut-down. The proximal tibia and distal femur are recommended sites. In an emergency, particularly if you are inexperienced, the central venous route is not recommended.

Reassess the circulatory signs and measure the **pulse** and **blood pressure after treatment** has been initiated. Tachycardia is an important marker of hypovolaemia. Hypotension precedes bradycardia which is a late sign in haemorrhagic shock, indicating an impending cardiac arrest.

A good response to the treatment of shock will reduce the tachycardia, increase the pulse pressure, improve peripheral perfusion, improve conscious level, raise blood pressure and increase **urine output**. A urinary catheter will therefore be required.

Subsequent fluid treatment depends on the response to the first fluid bolus. The **observations** described above must be repeated. If all haemodynamic parameters stabilize, haemorrhage has probably stopped. If not, repeat the fluid bolus and obtain an urgent surgical opinion. If this second bolus has little or no effect, commence blood transfusion with packed red cells at 10 ml kg^{-1}. Grouped blood can be available in 10 min and may be given while a full crossmatch (taking about 45 min) is prepared. If blood is needed, assume that emergency surgery will be required.

Disability

'Disability' refers to a rapid assessment of the coma level and the pupils.

- Is the child **alert**, **responsive to voice**, **responsive to pain** or **unresponsive** (the **AVPU** scale)? This is a quick and reliable way to assess coma. The Glasgow coma scale score can be calculated later, in the secondary survey.

- Assess **pupil size** looking for asymmetry and speed of **reactivity** to light. A sluggish response to light is the first indicator of brain dysfunction. Asymmetry of pupil size is found in 10% of the population; a difference of up to 1 mm is within the normal range. A greater discrepancy, particularly when consciousness is impaired, suggests intracranial pathology.

These brief neurological assessments, when repeated frequently, help to identify central nervous system deterioration.

Exposure

Undress the child to allow a full examination but cover areas that are not being inspected at the time. This helps to keep the child warm, to reverse shock, and maintains dignity in the conscious patient. The smaller the child, the greater the susceptibility to heat loss.

This completes the **primary survey** and **resuscitation** phases.

Investigations and monitoring

Radiography of the **cervical spine** (lateral view demonstrating all seven cervical vertebrae), **chest**, and **pelvis** is mandatory in all children with multiple injuries and the X-rays should be obtained as soon as feasible. Only if the child is stable should films be taken in the X-ray department, where better images are obtained than with a portable or overhead machine in the resuscitation room. The cervical spine view can wait as long as neck immobilization is maintained.

Radiographs of other suspected injuries are obtained later. More sophisticated imaging (CT scanning, angiography or ultrasonography) may be performed after consultation with relevant specialists and the X-ray department.

Regular monitoring of **oxygen saturation**, **capillary refill**, **ECG**, **blood pressure** and **other vital signs** is essential.

Baseline **arterial blood gas** values are needed, especially when respiratory problems are encountered, or consciousness is impaired.

Urine output is the best monitor of circulatory adequacy. A urine bag may be adequate but catheterization gives a more accurate picture. Catheterization in boys is contraindicated when there are signs of urethral trauma such as blood at the urethral meatus or a scrotal haematoma. The ideal output is 1 ml kg^{-1} h^{-1} in children and 2 ml kg^{-1} h^{-1} in infants. If there is a renal tract injury, urine output is unreliable.

A **nasogastric tube** will decompress the stomach. This is particularly helpful as acute gastric dilatation after injury is common in children and it causes pain and distress. Pass the tube orally if there are midface injuries or signs of a base of skull fracture (see Chapter 14).

If the child should deteriorate at any time, always **reassess** using the ABC sequence as described above. Failure to do this is dangerous and results in increased morbidity and mortality from potentially treatable hypoxia and hypovolaemia. Stay calm – if your mind goes blank, remember 'ABC'.

Secondary survey

Only begin the secondary survey when the primary survey is completed and the child is responding to resuscitation. Start the secondary survey at the head and work down to the toes. Make a full and detailed assessment of each area in turn, remembering to examine the back (by performing a 'log-roll') and inspect the perineum. Do not rush – the aim is to identify all injuries.

Head

Look for bruising, swelling, bleeding and other **signs of injury**, as well as **otorrhoea** or **rhinorrhoea**. Examine the **eyes**, especially the **fundi** and **pupils** (see Chapter 14). Follow guidelines for skull X-ray and CT scanning (Chapter 14).

Face

Look for bruising, swelling, wounds, deformity, bleeding and dental **injuries**. If the middle third of the bony skeleton is **mobile**, the airway is at risk of obstruction from the soft palate, so be vigilant if the child is not intubated. In small children, ask senior staff or the maxillofacial team for advice on X-rays as there is little facial skeleton and X-rays may be uninformative.

Neck

The head will need to be held and the collar removed for a full visual inspection and palpation of the neck. Manual immobilization must be maintained throughout this examination. The back of the neck and head can only be properly inspected during the 'log-roll'.

Look for **signs** of swelling, bruising, wounds and deformity. **Palpate** for surgical emphysema, bony tenderness or steps between the vertebrae.

Replace the collar and re-establish immobilization after the examination.

Chest

Re-examine the chest as described in the primary survey. Potentially severe, but not immediately life-threatening, **injuries** to identify include:

   pulmonary contusion
   simple pneumothorax
   great vessel, bronchial or oesophageal injury (mediastinum)
   diaphragmatic injury
   myocardial contusion
   rib fracture.

Bronchial and diaphragmatic injuries are more common in children but the major vessels are more resilient than in adults.

Fractures of the rib have a greater significance in children. Those of the upper three ribs indicate that major forces were involved and that the spinal cord, major vessels and other structures in the upper thorax are at risk. Further imaging to identify these injuries may be necessary, so seek advice.

Abdomen

Examine the abdomen carefully by **inspection**, **palpation**, **percussion** and auscultation. If the child is alert, follow the principles in Chapter 7. Insertion of a gastric tube deflates the stomach and can make examination much easier after the child has settled. Look for bruising, grazes and swelling, and feel for masses, tenderness, guarding and rigidity. Percussion is the kindest way to test for rebound tenderness.

Inspect the **perineum** but do not routinely perform a rectal or vaginal examination. Leave these procedures to the surgical team that will be looking after the child. If there are **signs of perineal injury** such as scrotal bruising, swelling or laceration, or blood is present at the urethral meatus, suspect trauma to the urinary tract and involve a urologist.

Emergency surgery is normally indicated when the shocked child has an acutely tender abdomen. **Referred pain**, for example to the shoulder, is an important symptom.

In other cases, **repeated examinations** are the key to successful detection of a developing pathological problem. These should be performed by a general surgeon if a paediatric surgeon is not available.

Diagnostic peritoneal lavage is rarely indicated in children; serial CT scanning, close monitoring and sometimes ultrasonography permit a more conservative approach to abdominal trauma in appropriately equipped units. Abdominal X-rays are rarely helpful, although supine or lateral decubitus films may reveal intraperitoneal air.

Pelvis

Palpate the bony pelvis, identifying **crepitus** and bony **instability**. X-ray of the pelvis will normally have already been performed. Haemorrhage from an unstable pelvic fracture can be lethal and associated visceral injuries may require emergency surgery.

Limbs

Inspect and **palpate** each limb, looking for **signs of bone and joint injury** such as tenderness, crepitus or hypermobility.

Assess peripheral **pulses** and **neurological function** distal to sites of any injury, especially fractures or dislocations. Most limb injuries can be repaired as long as the circulation is intact. Endeavour to exclude **signs of compartment syndrome** which is characterized by swelling and tenderness of the compartment, numbness affecting the compartmental nerve and pain on stretching the compartmental muscles.

Open fractures should be photographed with a Polaroid camera after any gross contaminant has been removed. The wound is then covered with an antiseptic dressing and the photograph is presented to orthopaedic staff, avoiding the need to re-expose the wound in a non-sterile environment. Commence intravenous broad-spectrum anti-staphylococcal **antibiotics**.

Radiograph sites of limb trauma as indicated. Growth plate injuries are common and may be difficult to diagnose without orthopaedic guidance.

Align fractures into their anatomical position and **splint** them to relieve pain, bleeding and shock. **Reduction** of fractures and dislocations is urgent if there is evidence of neurovascular compromise. Check pulses after any manipulation or movement of a limb and refer to the orthopaedic team.

Check **tetanus immunization status** and treat accordingly.

Spine

Three assistants are required to perform a co-ordinated 'log-roll' in a child (Fig. 23.2) leaving the examining doctor free to **inspect** the back for bruising, swelling or deformity, and to **palpate** the spine for bony tenderness and steps between vertebrae. This also provides a good

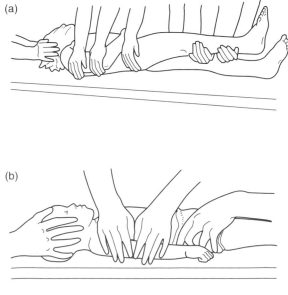

Fig. 23.2 *Log-rolling techniques.*

opportunity to examine the posterior ribs and the back of the head and neck by removing the collar if the head is held securely.

Remove debris, and any remaining clothing left on the trolley, before reversing the log-roll.

Request further spinal X-rays as indicated, particularly if the child is unconscious, the history involves falling from a height, there is any suggestion of thoracolumbar or cord injury from the examination, or cervical injury is confirmed. If you suspect spinal or spinal cord injury, SEEK HELP!

Nervous system

Assess the coma level using the **Glasgow coma scale** (see Chapter 14). Examine the **pupils** again, and the peripheral nervous system for **lateralizing signs** (unequal limb responses) or other **focal abnormalities**.

Check **sensation** and **power** if the child is conscious. Assess **tone** and **reflexes** for evidence of upper or lower motor neurone lesions and determine anal **sphincter tone** if spinal cord injury is suspected. Cardiovascular signs suggesting high cord injury are a relative bradycardia and moderate hypotension resulting from interruption of the thoracolumbar sympathetic outflow from the cord. Priapism is a rare but pathognomonic sign of spinal cord injury.

History

As the child enters the resuscitation room, only the basic **mechanism of injury** is important. *Focus initially on the primary survey and the sequence described above until you have control of the situation or a more senior doctor has taken over.* You can then be receptive to **detailed information** from the ambulance crew, relatives, witnesses and other emergency personnel. The **position** or **trajectory** of the casualty, **vehicle deformity**, **pre-hospital assessment and treatment** and **clinical response** to that treatment are some of the important factors to establish. Much of this information will be entered on the ambulance report form while you are resuscitating the child.

- Pointers to potentially serious life-threatening injury include:
    fatality at the scene

ejection from a vehicle
rolling or crushing of the vehicle
intrusion into the passenger compartment
high-velocity impact
fall from a height greater than 6 m
penetrating injuries (gunshot or stabbing) to the head, neck or
torso
- Children at particular risk of having a cervical spine injury include:
those involved in a high-speed accident
those with multiple injuries
those with any significant injury above the clavicles
those who are unconscious.

Reassessment

If no injuries are detected, re-examine the child as injuries may have
been missed.

FURTHER MANAGEMENT AND DEFINITIVE CARE

- **Analgesia** is important. Opioids should be given intravenously in
  the appropriate dose and titrated according to need. Inhaled gases,
  such as nitrous oxide and oxygen (Entonox), are not recommeded
  in serious trauma.
- Additional **investigations** will be selected by senior or specialist
  colleagues.
- Clinical records should be completed concisely, contemporaneously
  and accurately following the scheme described above. This will
  assist colleagues and help to avoid medicolegal problems. Non-
  accidental injury must always be considered.
- Surgery, intensive care, fracture stabilization and transfer to specialist facilities such as neurosurgery and plastic surgery will follow as
  indicated. Senior staff will arrange the transfer, the principles of
  which are listed in Box 23.1.

Box 23.1 *Principles of transfer*

Early liaison with surgical and anaesthetic teams is mandatory

Discuss the case with the receiving team and ensure that recommended treatments (such as mannitol in head injury or methylprednisolone in spinal cord injury) are completed

Organize transport as recommended by the receiving specialist

Arrange for a senior nurse and doctor to escort the child as appropriate – if the child is intubated or there are other airway or breathing problems, an anaesthetist is needed

Ensure as a minimum that ABC and resuscitation phases are completed and that the patient is stabilized as far as possible

Send copies of all notes and X-rays leaving none behind

Take a box containing all relevant drugs and equipment and be prepared for any eventuality

Keep the parents fully informed and offer a point of contact at the destination

Continue non-invasive monitoring at all times during the journey

If any deterioration occurs in the ambulance, stop at the side of the road to reassess rather than continue the journey

On arrival, give a detailed account of all that has happened from the time of the accident until arrival at the receiving hospital

OUTCOME AND PROGNOSIS

The approach advocated above and prompt attention to 'ABC' will significantly improve the outcome. Prognosis is a complex issue and is determined by the precise nature of the injuries.

24 NEAR-DROWNING

BACKGROUND INFORMATION

- 'Near-drowning' describes an episode of asphyxiation in fluid (usually water) followed by short-term or long-term survival. The term 'drowning' is used when the outcome is fatal.
- Near-drowning ranks as the third most common cause of accidental death in children in the UK (after road trauma and burns).
- An underlying medical condition such as epilepsy or diabetes may precipitate drowning, or there may be associated trauma if the child has dived into shallow water or has been hit by an object such as a surfboard or boat.
- The incident most commonly occurs in fresh water, and children playing in the vicinity of ponds, rivers and private swimming pools are at greatest risk. Most incidents involving children under 5 years old occur at home, and babies and toddlers can drown in the bath. Non-accidental events should always be considered.
- Children are prone to hypothermia because of their high ratio of surface area to weight, and hypothermia requires treatment in its own right. Although bradycardia, hypotension and shunting of blood to vital organs such as the brain may occur after submersion (the 'diving reflex'), hypothermia of rapid onset paradoxically confers most cerebral protection. Good-quality survival after prolonged submersion (up to 1 h) is only possible when the water is icy. For this reason, life support must be continued until core temperature is >30°C.
- About 10–15% of children die from laryngospasm with no post-mortem evidence of fluid aspiration.
- In the A&E department, junior doctors should never pronounce death on a child suffering from near-drowning or hypothermia. Such decisions must be taken by experienced doctors, and death must not be declared until basic and advanced life support have been continued, without success, for at least 30 min.

MANAGEMENT

Management in A&E is the same whether the incident took place in fresh or salt water.

Resuscitation

While the nature of basic life support provided at the scene of the incident is one of the most important factors influencing survival, the A&E doctor has to deal with the child in the condition in which he or she presents. A standard advanced life support sequence should be followed but as soon as notification is received, an anaesthetist and paediatrician (if available) must be called.

Airway with cervical spine protection

If the unconscious child has not already been intubated by paramedics, the airway must be opened, cleared by means of suction (use Magill forceps for solid debris) and then maintained using a chin lift and jaw thrust (see Chapter 19) until tracheal intubation can be performed at the earliest opportunity. Oropharyngeal airways should be used carefully as they may precipitate vomiting or regurgitation into an unprotected airway. Cricoid pressure helps to prevent passive regurgitation but is not safe during active vomiting. Maintain a head-down tilt until the airway is fully protected.

Unless injury to the head or neck can be excluded, ensure that an appropriately sized semirigid cervical collar is applied and cervical spine immobilization is maintained, or alternatively that the head is held in the neutral position.

Repeated suction may drain large amounts of fluid and debris from the airway before and after intubation. Pass a nasogastric (or orogastric) tube in the unconscious child to empty the stomach which is often full of fluid which may otherwise contaminate the airway.

Breathing

Before intubation, ventilate or assist ventilation with oxygen using a self-inflating bag and mask, avoiding high inflation pressures which will distend the stomach and encourage regurgitation. Following intubation, higher than normal inflation pressures and frequent tracheal suction may be needed. Intensive care is required when the child fails to respond promptly to ventilation in A&E.

Adminster high concentrations of oxygen using a reservoir mask in the child who is breathing adequately. Anaesthetic advice and care is necessary when the child fails to respond promptly to ventilatory support in A&E.

The conscious child should be encouraged to cough and clear the airway. Remember that vomiting occurs in over 50% of cases. Bronchospasm may be relieved by beta-2-adrenergic agonists nebulized with oxygen.

Circulation

Immersion and hypothermia both tend to produce bradycardia. The pulse may also be of small volume and the blood pressure unrecordable. A major pulse must therefore be felt for a minimum of 1 min before concluding that there is no cardiac output. Vascular access must be gained by means of percutaneous or intraosseous cannulation, or venous cut-down. Before any fluid or drug is administered, blood should ideally be withdrawn for routine tests, particularly glucose and electrolyte estimations. An ECG will have been applied and cardiac arrest or arrhythmias should be treated according to standard paediatric European Resuscitation Council protocols. If immersion has been prolonged, the child may paradoxically be hypovolaemic, as pressure from the fluid in which the child was immersed can reduce the intravascular volume. Hypothermia aggravates this hypotensive effect which may well necessitate cautious infusion of warm fluids.

Investigations

- Check blood results, especially glucose and electrolytes.
- All routine nursing observations, a Glasgow coma scale score and arterial oxygen saturation must be recorded regularly. An ECG should be monitored continously.

- A chest X-ray is essential once resuscitation is established, and sites of possible trauma such as the head and the spine should also be subjected to routine radiological examination.
- Monitoring of core temperature with a rectal probe, oesophageal probe or tympanic membrane thermometer is vital.
- Arterial blood gas analysis should be arranged as soon as resuscitation is fully established (blood gas values should ideally be adjusted for core temperature).

Management of associated hypothermia

The heart is irritable in severe hypothermia (core temperature less than 30°C) and undue movement or other stimuli can precipitate ventricular fibrillation which may not respond to direct current (DC) countershocks (or antiarrhythmic drugs) until the child's temperature is actively raised. The principles of treatment are therefore as follows:

- Manage the airway, breathing and circulation as described above. Hypothermia may cause stiffness of the chest wall requiring greater airway pressure for successful ventilation, and more forceful chest compressions to achieve the required sternal displacement.
- If core temperature is less than 30°C and ventricular fibrillation develops, obtain expert assistance to actively rewarm the child using appropriate fluid at 40°C circulated through the stomach (nasogastric tube), bladder (urinary catheter) peritoneal cavity (peritoneal dialysis catheter) and/or pleural cavity (chest drains). Inspired oxygen can be warmed in a humidifier and modest volumes of warm fluid may be infused intravenously. However, cardiopulmonary bypass is ideal if available.
- When the core temperature is greater than 30°C, the principles of rewarming are that children who have been immersed rapidly in cold fluid may be safely rewarmed equally rapidly (rewarming does not need to be restrained as in the elderly with urban hypothermia). The process should start with removal of wet clothing, drying to reduce heat loss through evaporation, covering the child with blankets and actively rewarming with an electric blanket or hot air duvet. Infants may be placed on a Resuscitaire. Bear in

mind that there will be proportionally greater heat loss from the head in small children and this can be reduced by using bonnets or other insulation.

- In mild hypothermia when the child is fully conscious, warmed, high-energy fluids will help. The uninjured, conscious child may also be safely immersed in a warm bath maintained at 40°C as long as this is comfortable and causes no sweating. Shivering should cease as the child rewarms.

- Administer intravenous glucose as necessary to maintain metabolism and heat production.

- Death cannnot be confirmed until the child is unresponsive to resuscitation after active rewarming to a core temperature greater than 33°C, or until attempts to raise the core temperature have failed.

Further management

Unconscious survivors will benefit from ventilation with continuous positive or positive end-expiratory pressure.

Steroids and prophylactic antibiotics have not been shown to affect outcome.

Even those children who appear to have made a satisfactory recovery from near-drowning must be admitted to hospital for observation. Secondary pulmonary oedema may develop.

The child who appears to have made a rapid recovery may be discharged after 6 hours if:

1. There are no respiratory symptoms such as cough or wheeze, nursing observations (temperature and respiratory rate) are normal and there are no abnormalities on chest examination.
2. Arterial blood gas tensions are normal on air and/or pulse oximetry remains normal.
3. The chest X-ray at this time is clear.

A full assessment for possible trauma should be carried out as described in Chapter 23.

OUTCOME AND PROGNOSIS

The heart is normally healthy in childhood, and as long as there is no irreversible hypoxic neurological damage the prognosis is favourable. Factors associated with death or permanent neurological disability are shown in Box 24.1.

   Of hypothermic children, the majority with reactive pupils and a third of those with fixed and dilated pupils make a satisfactory recovery. This confirms that fixed and dilated pupils cannot be considered diagnostic of brain death.

Box 24.1 *Factors associated with death or permanent neurological disability*

Delayed time to discovery of child

Prolonged submersion times (> 10 min; no survivors from *warm* water after 25 min)

Delayed or inefficient basic life support

Delay in the time to the first gasp (particularly if more than 20 min)

Failure to breathe spontaneously, or the persistence of coma, on admission to A&E

Core temperature > 33°C on arrival at hospital after immersion exceeding 10 min

Arterial pH less than 7 and arterial P_{O_2} less than 8 kPa

Prolonged advanced life support required (> 10 min – no survivors from *warm* water after 25 min, occasional survivors from *icy* water after 1 h)

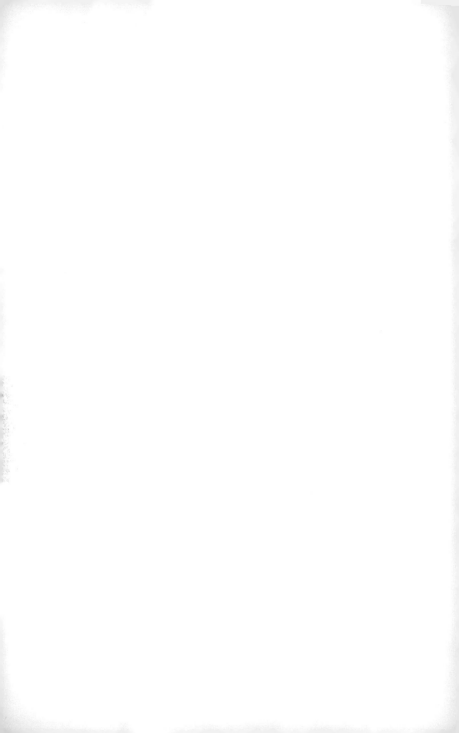

PART IV

Specific Management Problems

IV

25 MANAGEMENT OF PAIN

BACKGROUND INFORMATION

- The treatment of pain is frequently neglected in the A&E department.
- The inexperienced A&E officer may be unaccustomed to dealing with distressed, frightened children and may feel unsure about prescribing even simple analgesics.
- Experienced clinicians until recently withheld potent analgesics because of the widely accepted notion that children do not experience pain to the same degree as adults. Additionally they were worried about respiratory depression, cardiovascular collapse, reduced conscious level and possibly addiction associated with opioid use. Analgesia was given a low priority and children suffered unnecessary pain and distress as a consequence.
- The early assessment and treatment of pain will greatly improve the relationship that doctors and nurses will establish with children and their parents; it may help in diagnosis (since examination will be less distressing), and will be professionally rewarding.

IV

DIAGNOSTIC APPROACH

The assessment of pain can be extremely difficult and is dependent upon the interactions between the child's age or level of neurodevelopment, the psychosocial environment, and the nature of the injury.

Age

In the stressful environment of the A&E department children may regress to a more immature level of behaviour.

In children under 2 years old, pain assessment can only be made by observation of the child's behaviour, since they cannot tell you what hurts. Look particularly for crying or grimacing during examination. Is the child calm, rigid, thrashing, or showing localizing signs (e.g. pulling the ear or avoiding use of a painful limb)? How quickly does the child settle when comforted?

Some pre-school children may be able to localize painful areas verbally or by pointing, and can give some indication of the severity of their pain by using simple visual analogue scales such as the 'smiley face' or verbal rating ('Is it a little hurt or a big hurt?').

Schoolchildren are more sophisticated and can describe what hurts and indicate the severity. A verbal analogue scale of 0–10 may be useful.

Psychosocial factors

Pain and discomfort can only be assessed once the basic needs of food, warmth, a clean, dry nappy and a friendly environment (usually the presence of the parent) have been met.

The A&E department can be a frightening and intimidating place for children. They may be kept waiting, separated from their parents (though this should be avoided), denied food or drink, and toddlers may have their bedtime disrupted.

Increasing age and insight alter the child's response to A&E. Simple explanations can dispel some fears for parents and children alike.

Parents may have feelings of guilt, helplessness and anger, and they too are often tired, hungry and frustrated. These feelings reduce their tolerance and that of their child. A timely and sensitive explanation of what is happening, in an area designed for children, will make the requirement for analgesia easier to assess.

Nature of the injury

The severity and nature of the pain cannot always be gauged by the appearance of the affected part. Causes of pain may be hidden (e.g. acute otitis media). The ability to assess improves with experience and by listening to and observing the child and parent.

MANAGEMENT AND REFERRAL

Children – and nurses – hate intramuscular injections, therefore avoid them if at all possible. Syringes, needles and ampoules should be kept out of sight. Intramuscular injections should never be used in hypovolaemic patients.

Explain to the child and parent what you are going to do and why. Do not say a procedure is not going to hurt if it obviously will – you will lose the confidence of the child.

Prevention of pain is very important, so if time allows use local anaesthetic cream before inserting intravenous cannulae. Use local anaesthesia topically, by infiltration or a specific nerve block before suturing wounds or manipulating a fractured femur.

Simple physical methods of analgesia are often the most effective and have the least side-effects (see below).

Inhalation of nitrous oxide and oxygen (Entonox) gives excellent reversible analgesia especially for short procedures, e.g. manipulation of a fracture or dislocation. It is appropriate when the child is old enough to co-operate with its use.

Opioids are safe and effective if the child is under observation. Oral sedatives should not be combined with opioids unless given by an anaesthetist or senior A&E doctor with anaesthetic skills. Do not withhold analgesia because of an acute abdomen or head injury, but consult the relevant specialist. Calculate all drug doses according to weight (although this may have to be an estimated weight in A&E).

Some of the techniques required are specialist skills. For these, referral to senior A&E or anaesthetic staff is indicated.

Methods of analgesia

Simple physical techniques

The definitive treatment of an injury is usually the most effective form of analgesia. Examples include:

- Reduction and immobilization of a fracture or dislocation.
- Evacuation of a subungual haematoma or drainage of a paronychia.
- Application of a burn dressing.

Temporary measures include inflatable splints, ice packs, elevation of sprains and cold water on burns and scalds. Many procedures are painful in themselves and require prior analgesia, as described below.

Nitrous oxide

Entonox is a 50:50 mixture of nitrous oxide and oxygen which provides reversible pain relief of rapid onset suitable for short but painful procedures such as manipulations. It is administered through a demand valve to either a mask (preferably the clear silicone rubber type) or a mouthpiece that the child can bite on. Even children 3–4 years old can pretend to be fighter pilots and use the face-mask with very little encouragement. The demand valve can be raised by the doctor or nurse so that a constant flow is generated if the child has difficulty triggering the mechanism. The child should breathe the mixture for approximately 1 min until slightly dysphoric and lightheaded before the manipulation is completed. The technique can also be used to supplement other analgesia.

Nitrous oxide will not produce hypotension and it increases inspired oxygen levels. It rapidly diffuses into enclosed gaseous spaces, increasing the volume of a pneumothorax or obstructed bowel.

Local anaesthesia

Local anaesthesia can produce satisfactory, reversible analgesia (for example, to assist reduction of a fractured femoral shaft) without the systemic effects associated with the use of NSAIDs or opioids. This is particularly advantageous in a child with other major injuries since there will be no depression of conscious level, or of respiratory or renal function.

More commonly, local anaesthesia is used for minor surgical procedures in the A&E department. There are large numbers of different types and preparations of local anaesthetic agents depending on which area of the body requires analgesia and for how long. Topical preparations are described in the next section.

In the UK, lignocaine, prilocaine and bupivacaine are the local anaesthetic agents available for infiltration or nerve blocks.

- Lignocaine is most commonly used and it acts for approximately 1 h.
- Prilocaine has a higher therapeutic index because it is extensively tissue-bound. One of its degradation products may rarely cause methaemoglobinaemia in susceptible children, or if the maximum dose is exceeded.
- Bupivacaine has a slower onset but much longer duration of action (4–6 h) and is suitable for a major nerve block. Unfortunately it also has a lower therapeutic index because of its adverse effect on cardiac conduction.

The maximum safe dose of each local anaesthetic agent is shown in Table 25.1. These drugs are sometimes combined with vasoconstrictors – normally adrenaline 1:200 000 (5 µg ml^{-1}) – to prolong the duration of action, increase the dose that can be safely administered, or to produce a bloodless field. Vasoconstrictors should never be used in regions supplied by *end-arteries* (i.e. the penis or digits) because of the risk of ischaemia, so their routine use is not recommended.

The maximum dose in milligrams should always be calculated for the body weight of the child. Convert this to the maximum volume that can be used before starting to inject. A 0.5% solution is 5 mg ml^{-1} and a 2% solution is 20 mg ml^{-1}. Use the lowest effective concentration that provides adequate analgesia to reduce the risk of toxicity and increase the total volume that may be given. Suggested concentrations are:

IV

- Skin infiltration: 0.5–1% lignocaine or prilocaine.
- Nerve block: 1–2% lignocaine plus adrenaline, or 0.25–0.5% bupivacaine.

Hypersensitivity is extremely rare; however, toxicity will occur if the maximum dose is exceeded or the agent is accidentally injected into a

Table 25.1 *Maximum safe dose of local anaesthetic drugs*

Drug	Maximum dose (mg kg^{-1})	Maximum dose with adrenaline (mg kg^{-1})
Prilocaine	5–6	8
Lignocaine	3	7
Bupivacaine	2	3

blood vessel or into the cerebrospinal fluid. The needle should therefore be aspirated if the injection is given into a single site, and signs of systemic toxicity sought if large doses are injected close to major blood vessels. Toxicity initially causes central nervous system stimulation, restlessness, vertigo, tremor, convulsions, and then depression, coma and respiratory failure, followed by hypotension and cardiac failure or ventricular fibrillation. The latter is particularly resistant to treatment if caused by bupivacaine toxicity. Intravenous cannulation and resuscitation equipment are necessary when larger volumes of local anaesthetic solution are infiltrated more deeply, but not for routine suturing of minor wounds.

In the A&E department, local anaesthesia may be used in the following ways.

Topical anaesthesia

Lignocaine for topical use comes as a 2% gel or a spray (10 mg per dose). The gel is useful to anaesthetize the urethra prior to catheterization, as well as exposed tissues in localized abrasions or burns. The spray is normally used to anaesthetize the airway prior to intubation, and will provide analgesia for suturing the lip.

Emla cream (eutectic mixture of local anaesthetics) consists of lignocaine and prilocaine bases. It is supplied in 5 g and 30 g tubes. One or two grams should be applied per 10 cm^2 of skin and covered with a transparent occlusive dressing. Analgesia sufficient for venepuncture takes at least 60 min though it is less in children under 4 years old. It should not be used on dermatitis or eczema, premature babies, or children with potential methaemoglobinaemia (e.g. under treatment with sulphonamides, primaquine or nitrates). Emla cream can cause blanching of the skin and may make venepuncture more difficult if the veins are small. This is less of a problem with amethocaine. Ametop is a 4% amethocaine gel which produces analgesia of the skin within 30–45 min and lasts about 4 h. A mixture of amethocaine (tetracaine) 0.5%, adrenaline 1:2000 and cocaine 11.8% (TAC) is used in North America and is on trial in many centres in the UK for debridement and suturing. Its efficacy is comparable to infiltration with lignocaine but it achieves greater compliance. The components are potentially toxic.

Wound instillation and infiltration

Smaller needles (23 G or less) and warming of the local anaesthetic agent reduce discomfort. Dripping the local anaesthetic solution into the wound may be helpful. Small children may also require oral sedation before suturing (see below).

Nerve blocks

Nerve blocks are widely used in anaesthetic and dental practice. In A&E, the following are useful and safe in the conscious child:

- Digital nerve block.
- Femoral nerve block.
- Ulnar and median nerve block at the wrist (usually only by anaesthetic staff).

Some of these techniques are described in Part V. Other blocks (especially intercostal, epidural and intravenous regional blocks) may be performed in older children in the A&E department, usually by anaesthetists with an anaesthetic assistant.

Simple analgesics

IV

Paracetamol and non-steroidal anti-inflammatory drugs (NSAIDs) provide good analgesia for mild to moderate pain. They are usually given orally or rectally and cause no respiratory depression or impaired consciousness. Aspirin should not be given to children under 12 years old because of the association with Reye's syndrome.

Paracetamol is a palatable and effective antipyretic, and is extremely useful for treating both fever and pain (e.g. acute otitis media). It may be given rectally though the onset is slower and less predictable. In the past paracetamol has been given in inadequate dosage. Up to 30 mg kg^{-1} can be given as an initial loading dose with 20 mg kg^{-1} 6-hourly thereafter.

NSAIDs have anti-inflammatory properties and are particularly useful for soft tissue or bony injuries. They are as effective as pethidine for renal colic. They inhibit cyclo-oxygenase and therefore affect prostaglandin synthesis, which explains the majority of their side-effects such as gastrointestinal bleeding, platelet inhibition, asthma and reduced renal blood flow. They are contraindicated in hypovolaemia and bleeding disorders and should be used with caution in asthma. Table 25.2 lists the

Table 25.2 *NSAIDs used in children*

Preparation	Maximum daily dosage (mg kg^{-1})	Frequency	Dose (mg kg^{-1})
Diclofenac			
dispersible	3.0	8–12 hourly	1.0
rectal	—	12 hourly	0.5–1
(im painful – not			
recommended)			
Ibuprofen			
oral (elixir)	20	6 hourly	5.0
Indomethacin			
oral	3.0	8 hourly	0.3–1.0
Naproxen			
oral (elixir)	10	12 hourly	5.0
Ketorolac			
injectible	2.0	6 hourly	0.2–0.5
(iv/im)			

NSAIDs used in paediatric practice. Only diclofenac and ibuprofen are licensed for acute pain in children under 16 years (but over 1 year). However, the other drugs are used for juvenile arthritis, and ketorolac has been used extensively and safely for treatment of postoperative pain (e.g. after tonsillectomy).

Opioids

A large range of opioids is available; Table 25.3 lists the most useful agents for children in the A&E department. Ideally, no drug should be given intramuscularly to children. Intramuscular opioids are definitely contraindicated in hypovolaemia because initially they will be ineffective owing to poor absorption and then may have a profound effect once the circulation is restored.

Intravenous opioids should be given slowly in incremental doses to titrate to the desired level of analgesia and sedation. Naloxone 4 μg kg^{-1}

Table 25.3 *Opioids used in children*

Drug	Dose (mg kg^{-1})	Frequency	Indication
Codeine			
oral/im	0.5–1.0	6 hourly	mild to moderate pain
Dihydrocodeine			
oral/im	0.5–1.0	4–6 hourly	moderate to severe pain
Pethidine			
oral/im	0.5–2.0	3–4 hourly	moderate to severe pain
iv	0.25–0.5		
Morphine			
oral	0.2–0.5	4 hourly	severe pain
im	0.2		
iv	0.05–0.1		

should be available if large doses of intravenous opioid are required for analgesia.

All opioids depress respiration and conscious level when given at equianalgesic doses. However, codeine and dihydrocodeine in normal usage are less likely to cause respiratory problems. Opioids can cause hypotension and bradycardia especially in hypovolaemic patients because of the reduction of sympathetic tone when pain is obtunded. In addition, morphine may cause histamine release. All are associated with nausea, vomiting and constipation. Fortunately, nausea and vomiting appear to be less of a problem in children and so routine antiemetics are not required.

IV

Codeine

Codeine should never be given intravenously because it has been associated with cardiovascular collapse. It is used for mild to moderate pain, often in combination with paracetamol (co-codamol 8/500 is 8 mg codeine with 500 mg paracetamol, and co-codamol 30/500 is 30 mg codeine with 500 mg paracetamol). These are useful for dental or bony pain when NSAIDs are contraindicated. Intramuscular codeine (formerly used extensively for pain following neonatal surgery or head injury

because of its low potency) has been superseded by regional blocks or
NSAIDs.

Dihydrocodeine
Dihydrocodeine is more potent than codeine and an elixir is available for
children.

Pethidine
Pethidine is a synthetic opioid which may relax smooth muscle and
have a lower incidence of histamine release than morphine. It is thus
useful in biliary or renal colic and possibly preferable for potent analgesia in asthmatics. Repeated doses in chronic conditions such as
sickle-cell disease can lead to accumulation of the renally excreted
metabolite norpethidine. This may cause seizures, especially in renal
impairment.

Morphine
Morphine is the principal opioid for all severe pain in conscious patients.
The oral preparation Oramorph provides good analgesia and sedation
for children who do not require an intravenous cannula (e.g. for changing a burns dressing). In severe pain the intravenous dose should
be titrated, giving 50 µg kg^{-1} every 5–10 minutes until analgesia is
achieved. Maintenance analgesia with a patient-controlled device (for
children over 5 years) or a morphine infusion can be initiated in A&E, but
must be supervised by experienced nurses who can monitor sedation
and ventilatory levels.

Sedation

Distress in children results from fear in addition to pain. Sedation may
be required, especially if performing minor surgical procedures under
local anaesthesia. The child should be made calm and co-operative or
sleepy, but rousable to avoid aspiration or respiratory obstruction. This is
not easily achieved and some children may become paradoxically rest-
less and hyperactive. Sedatives must never be combined with opioids
because the effects are additive.

Contraindications to sedation are:

- Food and drink less than 6 hours previously.
- Hypoxia (e.g. airway obstruction, asthma, multiple rib fractures).
- Head injury.
- Hypovolaemia.

If a child will not tolerate a procedure after oral sedation, then help must be sought from anaesthetic colleagues.

Suggested oral drugs are midazolam 0.5–0.75 mg kg^{-1}, trimeprazine 2–4 mg kg^{-1} or triclofos 30–50 mg kg^{-1}. Midazolam has a very bitter taste but most children will drink it if flavoured with, for example, blackcurrant juice. Midazolam has the advantage of having a specific antagonist (flumazenil) which should be given intravenously in incremental doses of 10 μg kg^{-1} until sedation is reversed. It has a short half-life and sedation may recur.

Summary: Suggested analgesia

1. MILD PAIN: paracetamol or ibuprofen.
2. MODERATE PAIN: co-codamol (oral); diclofenac (oral/pr); dihydro-codeine.
3. SEVERE PAIN: iv opiates.

IV

SPECIFIC CONDITIONS

Acute abdominal pain

Analgesia was traditionally withheld from patients with acute abdominal pain because of the fear that it might mask the symptoms and signs. There is good evidence that this is not the case and if a child is made comfortable, a clearer history and examination may demonstrate localized signs. Intravenous opioids should be carefully titrated to produce a comfortable and co-operative child.

Head injury and major trauma

Minor head injury without a change in conscious level or skull fracture can be treated with simple analgesics. In severe head injuries, pain and distress will further raise intracranial pressure, so controlled sedation, analgesia and ventilation by anaesthetists is extremely important.

Difficulty is encountered with children who have some change in conscious level (GCS score 13 or below), other significant injuries and severe pain. A femoral nerve block and splintage will provide excellent analgesia and not cause sedation. Multiple rib fractures may be treated by the insertion of an epidural catheter and regional anaesthesia. Intravenous opioids can be titrated to achieve analgesia with only minor sedation. Patient-controlled analgesia can often be used thereafter. Regular neurological observations and access to a CT scanner are essential.

Burns

Burns and scalds are common in children. Intravenous opioids are the mainstay of analgesia in the acute extensive burn. Appropriate dressings will provide additional pain relief.

FURTHER READING

Lloyd-Thomas (1990) Pain management in paediatric patients. *British Journal of Anaesthesia* **64**: 85–104.

Illingworth KA & Simpson KH (1994) *Anaesthesia and Analgesia in Emergency Medicine*. Oxford University Press.

Nahata MC *et al.* (1984) Acetaminophen accumulation in paediatric patients with repeated doses. *European Journal of Clinical Pharmacology* **27**: 57–59.

Salter RH (1985) Diagnosis before treatment. *Lancet* **I**: 863–864.

Attard AR *et al.* (1992) Safety of early relief for acute abdominal pain. *British Medical Journal* **305**: 554–556.

Peutrell JM & Mather SJ (1996) *Regional Anaesthesia in Babies and Children*. Oxford University Press.

26 MANAGEMENT OF NON-ACCIDENTAL INJURY

BACKGROUND INFORMATION

- All staff working in the A&E department dealing with children must be constantly aware of child abuse and alert to the possibility that any injury may be non-accidental.
- One child in 10 000 dies as the result of child abuse in the UK.
- Non-accidental injury or physical abuse is only one manifestation of abusive behaviour: children may suffer sexual and emotional abuse, or neglect, and several different types of abuse may co-exist.
- In this chapter, the person attending the department with the child may not always be the parent and so is referred to as the 'carer'. The person responsible for abuse is referred to as the 'perpetrator'.

IV

Child protection procedures in the UK

- Child protection procedures in the UK have been devised by social services, police, health and other agencies working together on Area Child Protection Committees. The aim of the procedures is the prevention of abuse and the protection of the child subject to abuse. The procedures also support staff by providing guidance.
- Every A&E department should have a copy of the local Child Protection Committee procedures, with which staff must be familiar.
- Part of the child protection procedure is the registration of children believed to have suffered or be at risk of child abuse on the Child Protection Register, held by social services. The A&E department should have a mechanism for interrogating this register routinely when young children attend.
- It is good practice to notify the health visitor or school nurse, as appropriate, of all visits made by children aged 0–16 years to the A&E department.

- Many A&E departments have a liaison health visitor who will examine the A&E records and discuss any children causing concern. Relevant information can then be relayed to the child's health visitor who may visit the family at home.
- The key to all child protection work is communication between the many professionals who may come into contact with the child. Good inter-agency communication could prevent a tragedy.

DIAGNOSTIC APPROACH

General background

- Is the carer **more worried about personal needs** (e.g. getting home quickly) than those of the injured child?
- What is the **affect of the carer**? Does the carer seem depressed? Parents can suffer isolation and stress which may predispose to non-accidental injury. Is the carer making unreasonable demands on staff, or conversely, indifferent to the injured child?
- Has there been **unreasonable delay** in seeking advice (remembering that many parents wait until the next day). Delay beyond 48 h would be unusual; in some studies it occurs in 30% of child abuse incidents but only 10% of genuine accidents.
- Does the **story change**, or is it **vague**? To detect this, free communication with other members of the A&E team is necessary.
- Children whose carers are involved in **domestic violence** are at greater risk of non-accidental injury. Any obvious signs of injury in the attending carer should be noted.
- Is the child on the **Child Protection Register**? If so, suspicion is increased, but if not, this is no reassurance. Most children subjected to non-accidental injury are not registered.
- Allowance must be made for differences in **culture**. Common sense and 'street wisdom' will prove valuable.

These features of abuse may be absent in a child who has suffered non-accidental injury: they are not sensitive indicators. Conversely, they may be present in children presenting with genuine accidental injury, and are not very specific. Use common sense in the interpretation of these factors.

As with all child protection work, communicate your doubts to a more senior colleague or social services if you are uncertain about the circumstances.

History

- Obtain a detailed history about the **events leading up to the injury**. Where were the carers and why? Taking a little time to gather this information pays dividends. Genuine accidents tend to sound 'real', although sometimes unusual. By taking a detailed history, inconsistencies may appear.
- You should always **talk to the child** and, depending on the level of understanding and ability to communicate, take due note of what is said. It is unlikely, however, that a child sitting on the lap of some-body who has injured them will feel able to disclose the truth, especially if returning home with the perpetrator. It may be useful to **speak to the child alone**, but there are practical difficulties in a busy A&E department. A play area with a nursery nurse may provide a suitable environment for the child to speak out.
- From the **age** and **developmental level**, consider whether or not it is possible for the child at the time of the injury to have been doing what is claimed. A newborn baby will not roll off a bed. A child who is not yet walking is unlikely to fracture a leg.
- Do not forget the **social history**, paying particular attention to any **siblings**. Think of family stresses that may be reflected by parents, the child or the social background:

  the *parent* may be young, lack family support or have been abused as a child (incidence 20 times as high in these circumstances)

  the *child* may have been unwanted, 'difficult' (e.g. constantly crying) or 'different' (e.g. with special needs or learning difficulties)

  social factors include loss of work, loneliness or isolation, or a crisis relating to housing

- Ask to see the **Child and Parent-held Record**. Many districts issue these to newborn children and a substantial proportion of children under 5 years old will have such a record. It can provide valuable

IV

information on growth and development as well as previous attendances at A&E departments and other medical contacts (assuming
that the practitioners concerned have written in the record). Of
course the carer may not have brought the record: this can be
inadvertent or deliberate.

Examination

Examination has been covered in other parts of this book; the key sup-
plementary part of the examination when considering non-accidental
injury is to think about the **aetiology**. Could the injury have been
caused in the manner described?

- Ensure that there is no objection to your carrying out the examination. This would normally be from a parent, but in an emergency
  a carer may give consent. Remember that consent is also required
  from a young person of sufficient understanding: in a normal child,
  this is from the age of 10 years.
- Start with **observation** of the child and the relationship with the
  carer. Does the child look anxious or relaxed? The so-called 'frozen
  watchfulness' of chronic abuse is rare (and occurs late), but unease
  should alert you.
- Proceed to a **full examination of the whole child**, done in a sensitive manner so as not to upset the child and lose co-operation.
  Examine each part of the body and replace the relevant piece of
  clothing before moving on. Look in the mouth and under the
  nappy. Record all injuries, their position, shape, measurements and
  appearance. The use of pre-printed topographic charts can make
  this simpler.
- Certain injuries raise the index of suspicion for non-accidental
  injury. Characteristic features are outlined in the following sections. Some injuries are considered pathognomonic of non-accidental injury. It is rarely possible to be absolutely sure about how
  an injury was caused, but with experience it is often possible to
  give the balance of probabilities. This level of proof can be used by
  social services to protect the child. If you are not happy with the
  explanation, communicate your doubts to a senior colleague or
  social services.

Cuts and bruises

Parts of the body that stick out or have little subcutaneous tissue tend to bruise easily. Bruising on protected areas such as the inner aspects of the thighs or upper arms is much less likely to have occurred accidentally.

Be aware of common accidental patterns of bruising. A row of bruises of differing ages on each shin in an ambulant child is a normal finding. It is very easy for a 2-year-old to bump into furniture and bruise the forehead. Be on the look-out for cuts and bruises with unusual appearances, for example straight edges, imprints or artefacts. These are unlikely to be accidental.

Features that may help to distinguish accidental from non-accidental bruising are outlined in Table 26.1.

- Two black eyes are hardly ever accidental unless there is a basal skull fracture involving the anterior cranial fossa following an RTA.
- In finger bruises, blood is forced out from the underlying vessels producing a 'halo' appearance. Lash marks may display a cut with bruising either side. Slap marks may leave parallel linear marks.
- Human bite marks are crescentic whereas animal bites tend to be U-shaped. The intercanine distance is > 3 cm in the bite of an adult or child over 8 years. The marks from animal canine teeth may be prominent. In cases of doubt, dental impressions can provide proof of origin.
- Generally, bruises aged 24 h or less are red/purple; if there is a yellowish/brown discoloration, they are more than 24 h old. More accurate dating is difficult and requires expertise.
- Do not confuse a Mongolian blue spot for bruising.

Table 26.1 *Distinguishing accidental from non-accidental bruising*

May be accidental	May be non-accidental
Lower limbs	Trunk
Forehead in toddlers, distal to elbow and knee	Lower back, head, neck, buttocks, palms, soles and/or genitalia
If multiple, same age	If multiple, different ages
Rounded, vague edges	Sharp edges or bizarre patterns

Fractures

In non-ambulant children (roughly under 1 year old), about half of all fractures are non-accidental. Features that may help to distinguish accidental from non-accidental fractures are outlined in Table 26.2.

- Periosteal new bone formation and callus take 10–14 days to appear; a fracture showing periosteal reaction is at least 4 days old, and a fracture following birth trauma will have callus by 2 weeks.
- The sclerae in very young babies often appear blue, and with normal dentition, no limb deformity and no family history, the chance of osteogenesis imperfecta is less than 1 in a million. This possibility and other rare conditions require assessment by a paediatrician.

Table 26.2 *Distinguishing accidental from non-accidental fractures*

May be accidental	May be non-accidental
Single	Single but with multiple bruising
Multiple	Multiple and different ages
	Child less than 18 months old
	Multiple rib fractures – consider bone scan
Usually greenstick or transverse	Spiral or oblique
Involving distal limb	Involving proximal limb
Single, linear, narrow, parietal skull fracture	Multiple or depressed skull fractures
	Associated intracranial injury
	Complex, wide (or growing) skull fractures
	Spinal injuries
	Periosteal reaction from fracture not visible on X-ray
	Metaphyseal or epiphyseal injuries following traction or rotation

- Subdural haematomas may occur without a skull fracture – look for retinal haemorrhages.
- Falls from furniture less than 1 m in height (even onto a hard surface) rarely cause fractures.
- Epiphyseal injuries are classically caused by tugging or swinging a child by the limb, but can also be caused by shaking.
- Head banging does not cause skull fractures.

Burns

Children, like adults, reflexly withdraw from hot objects unless they have anaesthesia, are incapable of movement or are prevented from moving away. Burns and scalds are discussed in Chapter 18.

Features that may help to distinguish accidental from non-accidental burns are outline in Table 26.3

- Cigarette burns are uncommon; they are deep and circular with a central crater and raised edge; there may be charring and ash. Circular burns do not result from brushing against a lighted cigarette; such burns are triangular and superficial. Lesions such as impetigo have been mistaken for cigarette burns.
- The centre of the buttocks, in contact with the cooler surface of the bath, may be spared if a child is forcibly immersed in hot water. Similarly, the sole of the foot may be spared in a deliberate dunking of the lower limb.
- The palm of the hand tends to be burnt more commonly than the dorsum in accidents. For example, if the hand is deliberately held under the hot tap, the dorsum of the hand may be burnt.

IV

Table 26.3 *Distinguishing accidental from non-accidental burns*

May be accidental	May be non-accidental
Involving the upper body, shoulders or arms	Involving the face, head, perineum, buttocks, legs, hands and feet
Irregular outlines with splash marks	'Glove' and 'stocking' distribution
	Clear-cut demarcation line
	No splash marks

Petechiae

Petechiae are sometimes present on the face, neck and/or conjunctivae from attempted smothering. Otherwise they can occur in a limb distal to a constriction force, or from bruising.

Retinal haemorrhages

These occur in 80% of cases of shaken baby syndrome. They do not occur in cardiopulmonary resuscitation and occur in less than 3% of severe accidental trauma. They occur in 30% of deliveries but have all disappeared by 6 weeks. They can be unilateral in NAI.

Internal damage

Internal damage may include a ruptured viscus (e.g. liver, spleen) which may present as shock. Intracranial haemorrhage can mimic sepsis, with a bulging fontanelle.

Poisoning

Unexplained symptoms may result from deliberate administration of drugs or other poisons. The child may be moribund with signs of encephalopathy or liver failure.

Common substances that may be administered are tricyclic anti-depressants, salicylates, iron and salt. A notorious case involving the injection of insulin by a nurse shows that hospital staff are not above suspicion. The symptoms that may be seen are described in Chapter 9, together with supportive and specific therapy.

Investigations

Clotting studies, blood count and platelets

Consider taking blood for clotting studies, blood count and platelets if there is a large bruise or widespread bruising, and especially if there is bleeding from mucous membranes or a haemarthrosis.

Skeletal survey

A skeletal survey should be undertaken in a department experienced with this investigation. A 'babygram' (single view of whole infant) does not constitute a skeletal survey. It would be reasonable to consider a skeletal survey in all children younger than 18 months presenting with a fracture and in those under 2 years with extensive soft tissue injury. Discuss this with senior staff.

Bone scan

This is more sensitive in detecting rib fractures, undisplaced shaft fractures and subperiosteal haemorrhage, but the earliest time it can detect a fracture is 7 hours post-injury.

Photographs

These may be requested by the consultant but accurate recording of the injury in the notes is more important.

Toxicology

If deliberate poisoning is suspected, samples of blood, urine and vomit should be collected.

Other types of abuse

Sexual abuse

Sexual abuse is the involvement of children and young people in sexual activities which they are unable to comprehend, or to which they cannot consent because of their developmental immaturity. Most acts of sexual abuse leave no physical signs. Some that may present in the A&E department include a sore bottom, bleeding per rectum, sore penis, perineal tear or bruising, perineal warts, vaginal discharge, sexually transmitted disease, bruising or scratching on the inner thighs, and many emotional manifestations. The child may disclose sexual abuse, but this is unlikely in an A&E department unless efforts are made to facilitate such a disclosure. Remember that parental concern regarding the possibility of abuse may not be voiced openly and easily translates to anger.

Neglect

Neglect is the persistent failure to meet the physical, emotional and social needs of the child. It can include failure to protect the child from cold or starvation as well as failure to promote the child's health or development. The child may be dirty, infested with scabies or nits, have a severe ammoniacal nappy rash, or be inappropriately dressed for the prevailing weather. Children chronically exposed to cold may develop cold injury, with red, swollen extremities. The child may appear under-nourished and the height and weight may be below that expected, although a single measurement in the A&E department is not that helpful. It may be necessary to obtain past records from the health visitor or from the Child and Parent-held Record if available.

Emotional abuse

Emotional abuse is the persistent ill-treatment or rejection of a child which adversely affects both emotional and behavioural development. Such a child may be listless and uninterested, apprehensive, watchful or abnormally friendly.

Some parents make their child adopt the sick role: this is a variant of emotional abuse and has been called 'Munchausen syndrome by proxy'. The illness is unexplained and fails to respond to conventional medical approaches; the carer seems more interested in the effect of the condition on the medical attendants than on the child; the symptoms may be incongruous (for example, haematemesis in a well-looking baby), and they may only occur when the carer is around. In the A&E department, frequent attendances may provide a clue, but such children are frequently taken to many different hospitals.

MANAGEMENT AND REFERRAL

- *Think about the possibility of abuse and refer to a senior colleague or social services if you suspect child abuse may have occurred*. The correct person to refer to may be the head of the A&E department, a resident paediatrician, an on-call community paediatrician, or social services if you are an experienced practitioner. *Do not wait until the issue arises before finding out the referral pathway in your unit.*

- *Refer suspected sexual abuse early to a senior colleague, preferably a consultant paediatrician with experience in dealing with this issue.* If a further medical examination is required it should be done jointly by a senior paediatrician and police surgeon so as to minimize the number of examinations and ensure that forensic specimens are collected correctly.

- *Be honest without being confrontational.* Most carers will respond positively to a statement such as 'I am referring you to a more senior colleague because this is the procedure that has been set out and its purpose is to make sure that children are safe'.

- *Inform social services if the carer refuses to let you fully examine the child or walks out of the department.* In circumstances where staff believe that a child is at immediate risk of significant harm (e.g. where parents are threatening to remove the child from the ward, A&E department, or outpatient clinic), hospital staff must be prepared to contact a statutory agency directly and without delay. In extreme situations, the police service is the agency which is most able to protect the child, but the relevant social services department must also be notified (DoH, 1995a).

- *Keep good records.* These need to be fuller than routine A&E notes and time spent can avoid problems later. You may be asked to appear in court where good notes will be invaluable.

- *Write in the Child and Parent-held Record of the children that you see in A&E.* Whether or not you suspect abuse, this can be a valuable way of communicating with other professionals and it may allow a pattern of recurrent attendances to emerge.

What NOT to do

- *Do not allow the issue of confidentiality to prevent you from communicating your concerns to others.* 'Patients are entitled to expect that information which a doctor learns during the course of a medical consultation will remain confidential'; however, 'Knowledge or belief of abuse and neglect is one of the exceptional circumstances which will usually justify a doctor making disclosure to an appropriate, responsible person, or officer of a statutory agency' (DoH, 1995b). Health services and other bodies concerned with the care of children must co-operate to protect children; this co-operation may entail the disclosure of information which in other circumstances might be considered confidential. If there is reason to believe that a child is at risk, a doctor has the duty to disclose information so that effective steps can be taken to protect the child.

- *Do not feel that it is your responsibility to make a definitive diagnosis of child abuse.* This is difficult even for the most experienced doctors, and usually requires a period of investigation by a number of people. The lead agency in child protection is the social services department and it is their responsibility to investigate if there are reasonable grounds to suspect abuse. The role of the front-line doctor in A&E is to have a high index of suspicion and to alert others when worried.
- *Do not confront the carer with accusations.* This may be appropriate after fuller investigation but it is not warranted in the A&E department.
- *Do not mislead the carer* by saying that you are asking for a second opinion about the injury and its treatment. The real reason will soon become obvious.
- *Do not feel that the involvement of social services is a negative development.* Child protection procedures do not inevitably lead to the child going into care. Their aim is to keep children with their parents so long as they are safe. Sometimes parents need temporary support and social services are often able to provide this.
- *Do not admit the child if there is no medical indication.* A hospital ward is not a 'place of safety', but is a dangerous breeding ground for serious illness such as bronchiolitis and gastroenteritis. If you suspect child abuse but the injury is not so severe as to require admission, social services can arrange temporary fostering while investigating the case. This can often be with a member of the family, such as grandparents, with whom the child is safe and at ease.
- *Do not forget other children who may be at risk.* These may be siblings or children in the extended family to whom the perpetrator has access.

- *Do not carry out internal examinations or attempt to collect forensic specimens in cases of suspected sexual abuse.* This is a specialist task.

Orders under the 1989 Children Act

The following orders may be used by statutory agencies in the UK such as the police or social services to ensure the safety of children.

Police Protection Order

A police officer can take a child into police protection immediately for up to 72 h. This could be requested if, for example, a child is being removed from the A&E department and you believe they are at serious risk of harm.

Emergency Protection Order

An Emergency Protection Order may be used if the child is felt to be at immediate risk. It will usually be requested by the National Society for the Prevention of Cruelty to Children (NSPCC) or social services, and will be granted by a court if it is suspected that a child is suffering or is likely to suffer significant harm and that access to the child is required urgently. It can be valid for 8 days, with the possibility of an extension for a further 7 days.

IV

Child Assessment Order

A Child Assessment Order is used when the child is not immediately at risk but there is good cause to consider that the child is suffering or is likely to suffer significant harm, and the applicant believes that an assessment is required. The court will grant this for a maximum of 7 days and will stipulate how the assessment is to be carried out.

Written reports

If an investigation goes ahead, it is likely that the most senior paediatrician involved will prepare a report for social services and the court. You may, however, have to prepare a statement, so the following guidelines are suggested.

- *Reports must be confined to statements of fact.* Failure to do this could lead to some uncomfortable moments in court. If you give an opinion you are setting yourself up as an expert and the defence lawyer may well decide to question this if you are inexperienced. Hearsay (information given to you by somebody else) must be excluded from the report, or the source quoted.
- State who has requested the report. Give your full name and qualifications together with your occupation and an indication of your experience. State the date and time when you saw the child and give the circumstances. Name the person examined and any people who were present at the time and who provided the history. Detail the history and examination findings using language that would be understandable to someone without medical qualifications, and avoid technical terms unless there is an accompanying explanation. Give the results of investigations with a statement about their significance. Sign at the bottom of each page and keep a copy.

> Have a high index of suspicion for non-accidental injury
> Seek advice from more senior colleagues if in doubt
> Keep good notes

FURTHER READING

Meadow R. (1993) *ABC of Child Abuse*, 2nd ed. London: BMJ Publishing.

DoH (1995a) *Child Protection: Clarification of Arrangements Between the NHS and other Agencies*. Department of Health, Welsh Office. London: HMSO.

DoH (1995b) *Child Protection: Medical Responsibilities*. Addendum to *Working Together under the Children Act 1989*. Department of Health, British Medical Association, Conference of Medical Royal Colleges. London: HMSO.

27 MANAGEMENT OF UNEXPECTED DEATH

BACKGROUND INFORMATION

- Each year in the UK approximately 500 infants die suddenly and unexpectedly of sudden infant death syndrome (SIDS).
- In addition, each year approximately 500 children over 1 year old die suddenly and unexpectedly, mostly of illness or accident, and the needs of the families of these older children are very similar to those whose babies have died of SIDS (Dent *et al.*, 1996a,b).
- The dramatic reduction in the number of infants dying of SIDS in the years since the 'Back to Sleep' campaign in 1991 means that most health-care professionals (even those working in A&E departments) will have only very occasional contact with families bereaved in this way, and few will have much experience of caring for these families. It is therefore of particular importance that health-care professionals – especially those who are usually involved in the care of adults – are aware of the special needs of families whose child has died suddenly and unexpectedly. The aim of this chapter is to give information and insight into the special needs of these families both immediately and in the days and weeks after the death.
- To facilitate the care of families bereaved by the sudden death of a child, it is recommended in the UK that each health district should have a named health professional (usually a consultant paediatrician) with a particular interest and experience in sudden death in childhood (Blair *et al.*, 1996). This individual co-ordinates the care of the families, supports those in primary care and in the A&E departments, and acts as a source of information.
- Although the co-ordinating consultant paediatrician will usually become involved with the family in the provision of information and support shortly after the death of the child, it is most appropriate that the family receive their main bereavement care from people already known to them, such as their general practitioner or health visitor.

MANAGEMENT

On arrival in the A&E department

When notification is given that a child who needs resuscitation or who has died suddenly at home is being brought in, the A&E staff should prepare to receive the family. A nurse should meet the family and concentrate on their special needs, accompanying them from the ambulance to an appropriate area in the A&E department. Resuscitation should continue until a senior member of the medical staff (usually a consultant in A&E medicine, anaesthesia or paediatrics) decides that further intervention is inappropriate and that resuscitation should cease.

The question of whether parents could be in the same room as their child while resuscitation is continuing remains controversial. Some families have found it reassuring to know that everything possible was done and to see that throughout the procedure their child was treated with care and respect. Other parents have found the frenzied activity surrounding a resuscitation, and particularly the physical procedures undertaken, to be very distressing. Some health-care professionals (particularly if inexperienced) find the presence of parents or other relatives distracting and distressing during resuscitation. It is, however, important to be aware that parents may wish to be present and they should not be denied this opportunity. At all times the nurse who is not involved in the resuscitation is specifically responsible for the care and needs of the family.

Clinical responsibilities

The decision to withdraw or cease resuscitative attempts should be taken only by a senior and experienced member of the medical staff (almost always a consultant). Prior to stopping resuscitation, the senior doctor should talk to the parents, take as detailed a history as is feasible, and try to ensure that there are no known underlying metabolic or biochemical abnormalities that might be amenable to correction. It is important that parents are aware that resuscitation is continuing, and they should be informed of the worsening outlook prior to its discontinuation. The parents must then be informed that their child has died.

Routine samples may be indicated after death (e.g. full blood count, urea and electrolyte analysis, blood culture, blood ammonia, serum to be frozen for metabolic investigations), but other investigations can be done at the time of post-mortem (e.g. lumbar puncture, skeletal survey, stool virology). Discuss this with senior staff.

Invasive equipment

Considerable confusion surrounds the practice of removing or leaving in place intravenous or intra-arterial lines or tracheal tubes. If the lines were required for resuscitation, there is no concern about their placement, and it is not felt that the device contributed to the child's death (e.g. a pneumothorax caused by subclavian line insertion), such tubes and lines may be removed in the A&E department. This will be more acceptable to parents, and it is particularly important to remove tracheal tubes and intravenous lines in the neck which may interfere with the parents' ability to hold and kiss their dead child. If there is concern about tracheal tube placement, an acceptable alternative is to cut the tube off inside the child's mouth and then push it further down into the trachea (or oesophagus) so that it is no longer visible. The pathologist will still be able to ascertain where the tube was placed, but the parents will be spared additional trauma of seeing it.

The coroner and the post-mortem examination

It is important that at as early a stage as possible the most senior member of the medical team speaks to the parents and explains the need to notify the child's death to the coroner. When talking about the child it is very important to use his or her first name and to talk gently and sensitively, but to use the word 'dead' rather than euphemistic terms such as 'lost' or 'passed away'. It is important to explain to the parents that it will be necessary for a post-mortem examination to be carried out. The precise arrangements by which this is done will vary from place to place, but it is essential that the parents are fully informed of the local arrangements. It is important that the parents know exactly where the child is going from the A&E department. If this is to a mortuary in the same hospital then many parents will wish to accompany their child to the chapel or viewing room adjacent to the mortuary so that they can say their goodbyes. For many parents it is very important to be able to picture the immediate environment in which their child is being left and in which they will next see him or her.

Many families are distressed at the thought of a post-mortem so it is very important to explain to them that this will be done with care and respect. Many families have a distorted view of post-mortem examinations, gleaned largely from American films, and it is especially important to dispel these. Someone needs to explain that the pathologist is a qualified doctor who will examine the child, initially carrying out an external physical examination, some X-rays and perhaps taking some blood or other samples. The final stage resembles an operation. It is important that the family know that although tissue samples will be taken for microbiology and histology, the remainder of the organs will be replaced and the incision sites will be sutured. The child will be left with what resembles operation scars on the front of the chest and abdomen (usually sternum to pubis) and on the back of the head. It is important to reassure the parents that the child's face will not be disfigured and that they can see their child after the post-mortem, indicating that nothing has been done that medical staff do not want them to see.

An important aspect of discussing the post-mortem with parents is to make it clear that their consent is not being sought. The role of the coroner in all sudden and unexpected deaths, regardless of the person's age and background, should be explained, emphasizing that the coroner will order a post-mortem examination regardless of the wishes of the family or medical attendants.

Contact and follow-up arrangements

Before the family leave the hospital, they must be given detailed information on whom to contact and how, should they require more information or wish to spend time with their child. A clear and preferably written arrangement should be provided to answer the family's questions and to give more information, possibly about the post-mortem examination. It is often most appropriate for further contact with the consultant in charge to take place at the family's home with the general practitioner or health visitor, to ensure complete continuity of care and consistency of communication and information.

The role of the police

The parents must be informed that the police may wish to contact them and discuss the circumstances of their child's death. For sudden, unexpected deaths in infancy where there is no suspicion of trauma, poisoning or untoward actions by any carer, the history taken by the A&E doctor will normally be sufficient.

The way in which the police respond to sudden, unexpected deaths of children varies widely from area to area and is materially affected by the way in which the information is initially presented to them by staff in the A&E department. Sometimes the police will visit the A&E department or the child's home to obtain a statement from the parents, but this is uncommon when the features are characteristic of sudden infant death. However, it is important that the parents realize that asking and answering questions about the nature of the child's death as soon as possible after it has occurred may be painful but helps to protect the family from such questions or allegations later. The fact that a death is reported to the coroner does not mean that an inquest will necessarily be held, but again, practice varies widely from area to area.

Contacting the general practitioner

The family doctor and health visitor should be contacted preferably before the family has left the A&E department. This will facilitate arrangements for the joint home visit in a day or two. Most general practitioners will wish to make contact with the bereaved family, and they should be encouraged to do so as soon as possible.

Suppression of lactation

If the child who has died was a baby who was being breast-fed then parents should be given information on treatment of engorged breasts, which may include the prescription of bromocriptine to suppress lactation

Notifying the coroner

The coroner must be informed of the death as soon as possible, and in most hospitals the pathology department will also wish to be informed at this stage.

Debriefing

Finally, it is important that the staff involved find time for debriefing. An opportunity to talk with colleagues, even briefly, about the effects of the sudden death of a child may be very helpful for all concerned. The opportunity to do so again after a day or two may also be valuable.

The nurse's responsibilities

The environment

The family should be given a room and as much privacy as possible. Preferably the room should be one in which they can spend time either alone or with their child, not one in which there is medical or resuscitation equipment.

The family must be given the opportunity to spend time with and hold their child. Sometimes that may extend over several hours, and accommodation may have to be found outside the A&E department. Other families wish to leave soon after the death of their child, but return later – sometimes in the middle of the night. They should be reassured that this is normal and acceptable, and they should be allowed to do so.

Some families may wish to be present while their child is washed and dressed or may want to do it themselves either immediately or later, or sometimes after the post-mortem.

In discussions with the family always use the child's first name. Take photographs of the child and offer to do so with the family and child together. Hand- and footprints and a lock of hair are sometimes important mementoes which the families may wish to have immediately, or which may be kept in the medical records to be offered to the family at a later stage.

Follow-up arrangements

Give the family instructions on how to make arrangements to come and see their child. Make sure they realize that they may visit their child at any time of the day or night, but ensure that they know whom to telephone to make preparations.

One of the striking and unpleasant features for parents visiting a dead child is the extreme coldness of the skin. If a child is removed from the mortuary refrigeration for a half an hour to an hour prior to the parents' visit, the skin will not feel so cold, but pathological investigations will not be compromised.

Spiritual care

The parents should be asked if they wish to have a blessing or other religious ceremony and, if so, the hospital chaplain or their own minister or priest should be contacted.

Transport

Ensure that the family has suitable transport to take them home and that, if possible, a friend or relative will be with them.

Primary care team

Ensure that the family's health visitor and/or community midwife have been informed.

IV

The parents should be given an appropriate leaflet (e.g. *Information for Parents Following the Unexpected Death of their Baby*, produced by the Foundation for the Study of Infant Deaths), and put in touch with an organization offering telephone counselling (see list at end of chapter).

Finally, the importance of debriefing staff, as noted above, must be emphasized.

Future visits by the family to see their child

It is important that families are asked to give the staff at least an hour's notice. The family should be met at an appropriate place, close to the hospital entrance and accompanied by a senior nurse to the chapel. The parents should be allowed to express their grief in their own way. The shock and pain may make it difficult to absorb what is being said and therefore parents must be given detailed answers which may need to be repeated. The family may have difficulty making simple decisions which to them may be very important.

Discuss with the family what they would like their baby or child to be dressed in, and give the parents the opportunity to assist with this. For some families cleaning and dressing the child after the post-mortem is an important affirmation that their child has not been unnecessarily mutilated. For others, the sight of the post-mortem incision is especially distressing.

Ask the family if there are any special toys, pictures or belongings that they would like to leave with their child. Such possessions and toys must be treated with great care and remain with the child.

Parents may be uncertain about bringing siblings to see the dead child. They should be reassured that this will not be harmful if it is done in a loving and caring way and is considered part of the process of saying goodbye. In some ways, death is more frightening to adults than to young children to whom the concept of finality is entirely alien. Many children of 3–5 years of age may be helped in their understanding of the process of death by the opportunity to visit the dead sibling, and the fantasies of many older children can be resolved. However, no pressure should be applied to do this.

A detailed record should be kept of each visit to improve support, continuity and consistency.

Administrative arrangements

The coroner will issue a death certificate after the post-mortem examination and the parents will be required to register the death in the usual way. Once this has been carried out a funeral director may remove the child from the hospital mortuary to the chapel of rest.

Many funeral directors are very knowledgeable and helpful in making families aware of the options available concerning funerals. They may be familiar with particular religious or cultural traditions and many offer low-cost funerals for children. In the UK, families in receipt of income support, family credit, disability working allowance, housing benefit or council tax benefit may be eligible for a payment from the Social Fund to help towards the cost of the funeral. A list of helpful leaflets is given at the end of this chapter. It is useful if staff can give some guidance on the various options available locally.

Families should be made aware that it is usually possible for the child to be returned to their home either overnight or on the day of the funeral. This is sometimes a particularly appropriate time for friends, siblings and other relatives to visit and say their final goodbyes.

Most hospitals will have a bereavement support officer who should be well informed on these and other administrative matters, and should be available to provide information to staff and families.

REFERENCES AND FURTHER READING

Dent A, Condon L, Blair P & Fleming PJ (1996a) A study of bereavement care after a sudden and unexpected death. *Archives of Disease in Childhood* **74**: 522–526.

Dent A, Condon L, Blair P & Fleming PJ (1996b) Bereaved children – who cares? *Health Visitor* **69**: 270–271.

Blair P, Fleming PJ, Bensley D *et al.* (1996) The SUDI case-control study. In: *Annual Report for 1994 of the National Advisory Body for CESDI.* London: Department of Health.

Foundation for the Study of Infant Deaths. Leaflet entitled *Information for Parents Following the Unexpected Death of Their Baby* by PJ Fleming.

IV

HELPLINES

Foundation for the Study of Infant Deaths
14 Halkin Street
London, SW1X 7DP
24-hour Cot Death Helpline: 0171 235 1721

Compassionate Friends
53 North Street
Bedminster
Bristol BS3 1EM
Helpline: 0117 953 9639

Child Death Helpline: 0800 282 986
Every evening 7.00 pm to 10.00 pm and Wednesday 10.00 am to 1.00 pm

SOCIAL SECURITY LEAFLETS

D49 *What to Do after a Death in England and Wales*
SB16 *A Guide to the Social Fund*
SFL2 *How the Social Fund can Help You*

PART V

Practical Procedures and Fracture Management

V

28 PRACTICAL PROCEDURES

This chapter is concerned with practical aspects of the management of children in the A&E department. The following procedures are described:

1. Incision and drainage of abscesses.
2. Aspiration of joints.
3. Needle cricothyrotomy and surgical cricothyrotomy.
4. Intraosseous access and infusion.
5. Cut-down procedures.
6. Venepuncture.
7. Suprapubic aspiration.
8. Nasogastric tube insertion.
9. Spacer devices and inhaler techniques.
10. Removal of foreign body from ear or nose.
11. Femoral nerve block.

V

1. INCISION AND DRAINAGE OF ABSCESSES

INDICATIONS

An abscess is a collection of pus which has been walled off by the body. It requires drainage, not antibiotics which will not penetrate the abscess wall. Lymphangitis and nodal spread are treated with antibiotics, and these are also appropriate for indurated areas where there is no evidence of suppuration.

CONTRAINDICATIONS

General anaesthesia (usually outside the A&E department) is indicated for:

    large or multiple abscesses
    abscesses in sensitive areas
    children too young to co-operate with local anaesthesia

Incision and drainage are only recommended when there is good clinical evidence of suppuration. In the older child, this can be confirmed by attempting aspiration of the lesion first.

Other contraindications to incision and drainage include inflamed swellings masquerading as abscesses (e.g. ganglia, false aneurysms).

EQUIPMENT

1. Sedative medication or other distraction technique
2. Means of immobilization (e.g. sheet for wrapping child, or several assistants)
3. Local anaesthetic equipment where indicated
4. Minor surgical equipment including a scalpel, dissecting forceps, sinus forceps and scissors
5. Small, plastic corrugated (Yeates) drains
6. Absorbent dressings

PRE-PROCEDURAL CHECKS

Arrange a stick assay or urinalysis for hyperglycaemia.

TECHNIQUE

Establish general or local anaesthesia although the latter may be only partially effective. Incise the abscess while covering it loosely with a swab to prevent dispersal of pus. Collect pus for culture, or take a swab sample if the lesion is small. In larger abscesses, break down loculations with sinus forceps or a small finger. Irrigate the abscess until all pus and debris has been released. In small abscesses, excise a narrow ellipse of skin to prevent premature closure of the abscess mouth. In larger abscesses, a small corrugated drain or similar device should be sutured to the wall of the abscess to prevent premature closure. Do not pack the abscess cavity as this will delay its closure, trap material in the base, necessitate painful changes of packing and increase scarring. The area needs to drain. Apply an absorbent dressing.

AFTERCARE

Initially, the absorbent dressing will need to be changed daily, especially if the abscess is large. Drains should be removed at 3–5 days, according to healing. Broad-spectrum (antistaphylococcal) antibiotics are only indicated for regional spread of infection.

COMPLICATIONS

Recurrent abscess formation usually results from inadequate incision and drainage. In paronychia small abscesses require incisions at least 1 cm in length (or a small ellipse). Provided the diagnosis of abscess is correct, complications are rare.

Some experienced staff incise, empty, irrigate and debride abscesses before closing them by primary suture under antibiotic cover. With careful technique, good healing with less scarring is achieved, but this approach should be left to experienced staff.

V

2. ASPIRATION OF JOINTS

Only two joints are amenable to aspiration in children: the knee and the elbow.

INDICATIONS

Significant joint effusions or haemarthrosis are the main indications. The aim is to reduce pain from joint distension and to improve the range of movement.

Any superficial joint should be aspirated if possible when the effusion is associated with symptoms and signs of infection (i.e. septic arthritis).

CONTRAINDICATIONS

The presence of a severe fracture or a wound at the site of the intended aspiration, particularly if the wound is contaminated, is a contraindication to this procedure.

EQUIPMENT

1. Local anaesthetic equipment
2. Assistance
3. Antiseptic (e.g. povidone-iodine)
4. Sterile gloves and drapes
5. Sterile 20 ml syringe and needle (normally 21 G)
6. Receiver for aspirate
7. Adhesive dressing
8. Culture vessel if joint infection suspected

PRE-PROCEDURAL CHECKS

Explain the procedure and its indications to the child and the family. Ensure that the child is appropriately sedated if necessary and that assistants have control so that the child will not jerk as the local anaesthetic solution is infiltrated, risking further injury.

TECHNIQUE

Use an aseptic approach. Clean the skin with antiseptic and drape off the area.

Infiltrate local anaesthetic solution (e.g. 1% lignocaine) at the site of intended aspiration. For the knee, this should be lateral to the upper pole of the patella, and for the elbow, midway between the lateral epicondyle and the olecranon. For sepsis in other joints, aim for the area of maximal joint distension. Infiltrate the local anaesthetic solution increasingly deeply until the joint is entered, as evidenced by the return of fluid into the syringe on gentle aspiration. Remove the syringe from the needle.

Apply a 20 ml syringe and aspirate blood or joint fluid. Apply gentle pressure to the opposite side of the joint to push the last of the fluid towards the syringe. From small joints, aspiration of just a few millilitres will relieve distension and pain. Only a few drops of fluid are necessary for microscopy and culture and when infection is suspected, immediate microscopy should be undertaken.

Seal the entry point with an adhesive dressing.

AFTERCARE

Arrange clinical review according to the underlying problem.

COMPLICATIONS

V

Complications are rare. Introduction of infection into the joint is uncommon as long as a correct aseptic approach is employed. Small joints should be approached avoiding neurovascular structures which can suffer partial injury (e.g. a neuroma). An unco-operative child may cause the procedure to become traumatic.

3. NEEDLE CRICOTHYROTOMY AND SURGICAL CRICOTHYROTOMY

INDICATIONS

The aim of cricothyrotomy is to rapidly establish access to the respiratory tract in the event of upper airway obstruction (resulting from trauma, an impacted foreign body or epiglottitis, for example). The main indication is a failure to secure the airway by tracheal intubation.

CONTRAINDICATIONS

Tracheal intubation should have been attempted if feasible.

The surgical technique is contraindicated in children below the age of 12 years, when the cricoid ring may be inadvertently divided (this cartilage prevents the trachea from collapsing in children).

EQUIPMENT

Needle cricothyrotomy

1. Assistants to immobilize the head
2. A standard 14 G cannula
3. A three-way Luer tap to connect tubing to cannula
4. Oxygen tubing with either a side hole cut in it or a Y connector in place to allow pressure to be realeased
5. An oxygen source

Surgical cricothyrotomy

1. Local anaesthetic equipment
2. Scalpel
3. Tracheal spreaders or curved mosquito forceps
4. Disposable cuffed tracheostomy tube (normally 6 mm internal diameter)

5. Self-inflating reservoir bag
6. Suture material and equipment
7. Oxygen source

PRE-PROCEDURAL CHECKS

Ensure that all the equipment is to hand before commencing and that the child's head and neck are controlled. In the absence of trauma, it is advisable to place a small pillow between the scapulae to extend the neck and expose the larynx.

Before performing a surgical cricothyrotomy a visor should be worn in addition to standard protective clothing.

TECHNIQUE

Needle cricothyrotomy

Attach the 20 ml syringe to the cannula. Locate the cricothyroid membrane in the midline between the cricoid cartilage below and the thyroid cartilage ('Adam's apple') above (Fig. 28.3.1). Insert the cannula through the centre of the membrane, directing it inferiorly at an angle of 45°, aspirating for air (Fig. 28.3.2). When this is found, slide the cannula forwards over the needle and down the trachea (as in cannulating a vein). Firmly connect a Luer connector to the cannula and attach the oxygen tubing, which needs to be trimmed to fit tightly into the Luer connector. Double the tubing over a finger and cut a side port in it before connecting the tubing to wall oxygen or a similar source. Turn the oxygen flow rate to the same number of litres per minute as the child's age (years). Ventilate by occluding the side port with a finger for 1 s and releasing it for approximately 4 s; however, it is more important to look for adequate chest expansion and to release the pressure before overexpansion occurs. Maintain these cycles until appropriate anaesthetic or ENT assistance is obtained – needle cricothyrotomy is only a holding manoeuvre. Ensure that help is on the way.

V

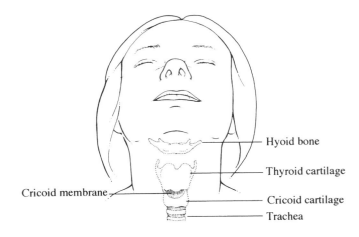

Hyoid bone

Thyroid cartilage

Cricoid membrane

Cricoid cartilage

Trachea

Fig. 28.3.1 *Anatomical landmarks for cricothyrotomy*

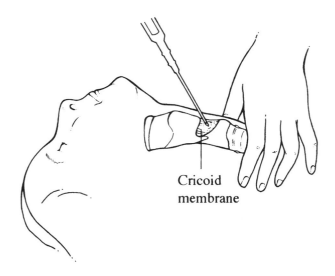

Cricoid membrane

Fig. 28.3.2 *Needle cricothyrotomy*

Surgical cricothyrotomy (Figs 28.3.3 and 28.3.4)

After positioning and stabilizing the neck, infiltrate local anaesthetic solution subcutaneously over the cricothyroid membrane if some ventilation can be achieved and a few minutes delay is permissible. If the child is *in extremis*, proceed immediately. The larynx must be fixed

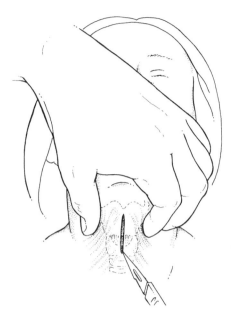

Fig. 28.3.3   *Surgical cricothyrotomy.*

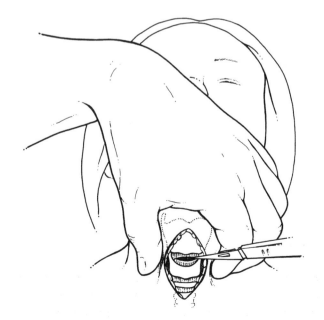

Fig. 28.3.4   *Surgical cricothyrotomy.*

firmly in position by the non-dominant hand. Incise the skin longi-
tudinally in the midline before rotating the blade transversely and per-
forating the cricothyroid membrane. Do not direct the blade upwards
in the direction of the vocal cords. Stimulation of the wall of the larynx will cause the patient to cough, spraying blood upwards, so a
visor is necessary. Insert the tracheal spreaders or curved mosquito
forceps through the wound and inferiorly, thereby maintaining patency
of the aperture and, hopefully, some spontaneous ventilation. Insert
the tracheostomy tube between the points of the spreader or forceps
which remain in place until the tube has been passed down the trachea and into position. Inflate the cuff and connect the tracheostomy
tube to a self-inflating reservoir bag connected to oxygen, ventilating
the child if respiration is inadequate. Maintain control of the tracheostomy tube until the side flanges are sutured in place. Auscultate
the chest.

AFTERCARE

In needle cricothyroidotomy, there is no egress of carbon dioxide
through the cannula – carbon dioxide is either retained in the pulmonary tree or it leaks out through the upper airway. Carbon dioxide
retention therefore develops at a rate dependent on the degree of
upper airway obstruction. The procedure buys time. An experienced
anaesthetist or ENT surgeon must be involved promptly after either
procedure.

COMPLICATIONS

- Local trauma to laryngeal structures, the oesophagus lying posteri-
  orly, vessels and nerves lying each side (e.g. the recurrent laryngeal
  nerve) can occur.
- There may be a failure to place the needle or tube within the
  trachea, resulting in continuing hypoxia and surgical emphysema
  during ventilation.
- Blood may track down into the pulmonary tree.
- Subglottic stenosis can develop after surgical cricothyroidotomy.

4. INTRAOSSEOUS INFUSION

INDICATIONS

The aim of intraosseous infusion is to achieve emergency vascular access in children, usually up to the age of 6 years, when routine percutaneous cannulation is unsuccessful. Blood can often be obtained by this route for emergency testing and crossmatch, and all standard intravenous fluids and drugs may be administered this way.

In cardiac arrest, intraosseous access should be established if percutaneous cannulation is not achieved within 90 s.

CONTRAINDICATIONS

Intraosseous cannulation should not be attempted on a fractured bone, or on a limb containing a significant fracture proximally.

EQUIPMENT

1. Assistant to control the limb
2. Skin cleanser
3. Sterile gloves
4. Local anaesthetic equipment
5. Intraosseous needle equipment. Various types are available: the smooth one is appropriate for small children and the threaded type for the older ones
6. Syringe for aspiration
7. The required fluid or drug for administration
8. Scalpel

V

PRE-PROCEDURAL CHECKS

Ensure good lighting and preparation of the equipment.

TECHNIQUE

Rapidly clean the skin over the surface of the tibia. If there is no immediate urgency, local anaesthetic solution can be infiltrated subcutaneously. One finger-breadth below the tibial tuberosity, make a small
nick with a scalpel in the skin over the centre of the subcutaneous
(anteromedial) surface. Insert the point of the intraosseous needle (with
trocar in place) directly through the stab wound onto the centre of the
tibial surface and keep it perpendicular (or pointing slightly inferiorly)
(Fig. 28.4.1). Apply pressure to the intraosseous needle as the trocar is
rotated. The smooth needle will suddenly breach the anterior cortex,
traverse the marrow cavitiy, and impinge on the far side. The threaded
needle must be rotated until it has passed into the marrow cavity. With
both types of needle, confirm communication with the marrow cavity by
successfully withdrawing blood or bloodstained fatty material with the
syringe (the trocar must be removed from the smooth needle first).
Finally, fit a three-way tap and connect the fluid or administer the relevant drugs using a syringe. Gravity flow of fluid is not always achieved
but fluid can be syringed through the needle using the three-way tap. If
the needle is unstable, consider suturing the flanges to the skin.

AFTERCARE

If a smooth needle is only being used intermittently, keep it clean by
reinserting the sterile trocar. Apply a large, soft dressing to protect and

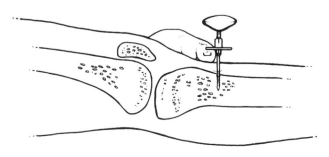

Fig. 28.4.1 *Insertion of an intraosseous needle.*

stabilize the needle, and bandage this in place. Aim to establish definitive intravenous access.

COMPLICATIONS

As the needle should only stay in until definitive vascular access is achieved, no significant complications are likely to result.

5. CUT-DOWN PROCEDURES

INDICATIONS

Cut-down procedures are used after failure to establish intravenous access, particularly in children over the age of 6 years in whom intraosseous cannulation is less successful.

CONTRAINDICATIONS

There is no contraindication of significance. There should be no wound or scarring involving the vein proximal to the point of intended entry.

EQUIPMENT

1. Local anaesthetic equipment
2. A range of cannulae
3. No. 11 scalpel and minor surgical equipment
4. Non-absorbable surgical ties
5. Syringe
6. Fluid or drugs for administration
7. Sutures
8. Dressings

PRE-PROCEDURAL CHECKS

At least one attempt at percutaneous cannulation should have been made.

Choose a vein. The safest site is the long saphenous vein lying 1–2 cm anterior to the medial malleolus. Other sites include the basilic vein over the medial side of the antecubital fossa, or the long saphenous vein below the medial groin, before it penetrates the deep fascia (this route is particularly useful when rapid infusion of fluid is required in hypovolaemia).

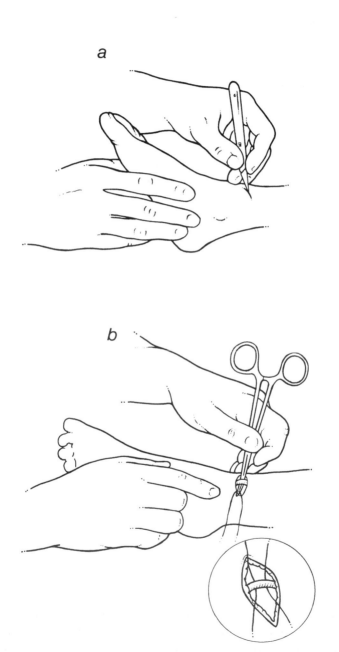

a

b

V

Fig. 28.5.1 a and b

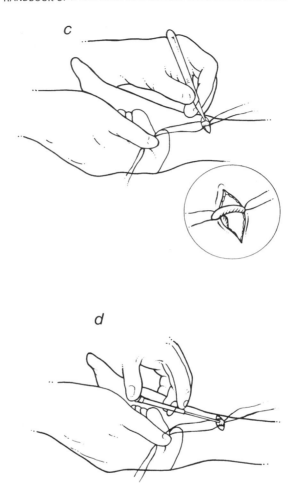

Fig. 28.5.1 c and d

TECHNIQUE (Figs 28.5.1 a, b, c, d)

If time allows, a small amount of local anaesthetic solution may be infiltrated in the area of operation.

After briefly cleaning the skin, incise transversely across the normal anatomical position of the vein, aiming to pass through the skin only. Dissect bluntly using mosquito forceps until the vein is seen, spreading the points of the forceps in the line of the vein to avoid transecting it. Insert curved mosquito forceps underneath the vein and pull a loop of suture tie through from the opposite side. Divide the tie to produce an upper and lower ligature. Ligate the distal end of the vein, leaving the suture long so that traction can be applied. With an assistant raising the proximal end of the vein with the other loop of suture, the wound aperture should be held open. Incise the vein from the side with the point of a no. 11 scalpel flicking the blade anteriorly so that the posterior half of the vein wall remains intact. Slacken the superior loop of suture material allowing blood to run back and the lumen of the vein to be seen. If necessary, dilate the lumen of the vein with fine forceps. Insert the largest cannula that the vein will accommodate *without its needle* (which may penetrate the posterior wall). Aspirate blood for any tests required. Connect the fluid or administer the required drug after tying the upper ligature to stabilize the cannula. Slightly close the wound by suture if necessary and stitch the neck of the cannula to the skin. Apply a sterile dressing.

AFTERCARE

The cutdown is likely to be temporary but the wound must be kept clean while it remains in use. On removal, the proximal end of the vein should be caught in a clip and ligated before the skin is sutured.

COMPLICATIONS

V

Infection sometimes develops, and structures adjacent to the vein (e.g. the saphenous nerve) can be traumatized.

6. VENEPUNCTURE

INDICATIONS

Any situation in which venous access or blood samples would aid diagnosis or treatment is an indication for venepuncture.

CONTRAINDICATIONS

There are no specific contraindications but care should be taken in individuals with known coagulation disorders. Try to avoid sites of obvious skin irritation (e.g. eczema) or infection.

EQUIPMENT

1. Skin cleanser
2. Local anaesthetic cream – lignocaine plus prilocaine (Emla) cream or amethocaine (Ametop)
3. Syringes – 2 ml, 5 ml or 10 ml
4. Needles – 21 G (23 G for younger children) or a butterfly needle; 19 G or 20 G needles may also be useful.
5. Tourniquet (particularly for older children) or assistance (for younger children)
6. Blood bottles (paediatric blood bottles if available)
7. Cannulae (if vascular access is also required)
8. Cotton-wool

PRE-PROCEDURAL CHECKS

Ensure all equipment is readily at hand and that the skin is clean. Explain the procedure to the child and carers wherever possible. If the situation is not an emergency, local anaesthetic cream can be used but it requires at least 30–60 min to take effect. Often the first attempt is the best, so ensure adequate help is at hand to restrain a young child as necessary.

An asistant often provides a better tourniquet by immobilizing the limb and permitting instant release at the correct moment.

Distract the child as you approach with the needle!

TECHNIQUE

The selection of the venesection site is a personal choice but the following guidelines can be used:

1. Age > 2 years: the antecubital fossa can often be successfully used. Alternatives include veins on the back of the hand or foot.
2. Age < 2 years: venesection is often easier on the dorsum of the hands or feet. A butterfly needle can be used, or (in more difficult cases), the hub of a 20G needle may be broken off and the needle passed through the skin along the line of a vein. Once punctured, the blood will drip through the end of the needle. (*Note*: ALTHOUGH THIS PROCEDURE IS COMMONLY USED, THE MEDICAL DEFENCE UNIONS WARN THAT DOCTORS CANNOT BE DEFENDED IF A COMPLICATION DEVELOPS, I.E. FIND YOUR NEEDLE!)

Occasionally venesection is difficult (in which case senior help should be sought) but a heel-prick sample from a small baby may yield enough blood for an FBC and U&E estimation but haemolysis is not uncommon.

In most laboratories only small samples are needed and paediatric blood containers are usually available for this purpose. Typically, many of the standard tests (e.g. FBC, U&E) can be performed on quantities less than 0.5 ml.

In an unwell child, an intravenous cannula should be sited immediately and blood can be obtained from the end of the cannula.

1. For a cannula 22 G or over this can be done by placing the syringe on the end of the cannula and withdrawing.
2. For a smaller cannula (24 G), two options are available:
    the blood can be allowed to drip from the end of the cannula directly into the bottles, or
    a 2 ml syringe with an orange needle attached (25 G) can be used to slowly withdraw a small amount of blood from the cannula end. This will also obtain a good uncontaminated sample for blood culture.

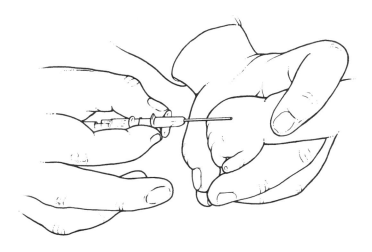

Fig. 28.6.1 *Cannulation of an infant*

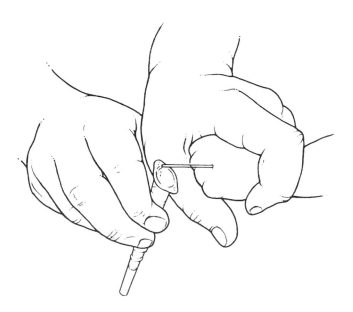

Fig. 28.6.2 *'Broken needle' technique.* (Note: **See Medical Defence Union warning in text**)

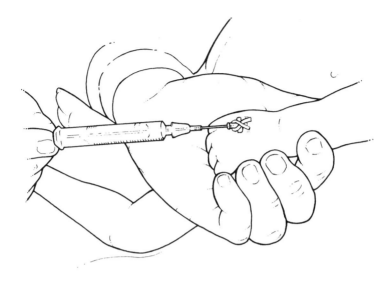

Fig. 28.6.3 *Aspirating blood from a cannula*

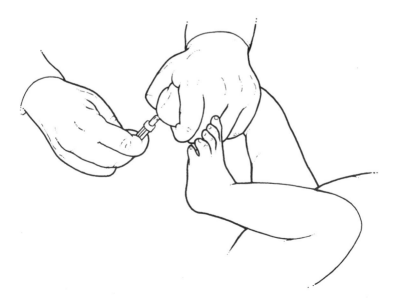

V

Fig. 28.6.4 *'Heel prick' technique*

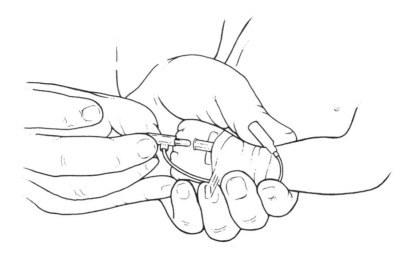

Fig. 28.6.5 *Extension 'T-piece'.* (Note: *may have Luer lock attachment.*)

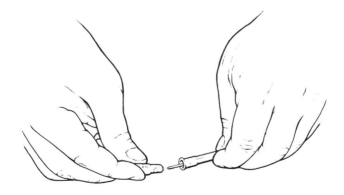

Fig. 28.6.6 *Breaking the hub off a green needle.* (Note: **See Medical Defence Union warning in text**)

AFTERCARE

Use cotton-wool on the venepuncture site after completing the procedure (alcohol wipes sting). Continuous pressure should be exerted over the venepuncture site for at least 1 min.

Clean off any topical anaesthetic cream at the end of the procedure (it can produce skin reactions).

COMPLICATIONS

- Failure. The first attempt will often fail. As a general rule, three failures should prompt the call for more senior help as further attempts will distress the child and ruin venepuncture sites. Consider alternatives where venous access is urgently required (e.g. intraosseous access or venous cut-down).
- Bleeding is usually preventable using the procedures described above.

7. SUPRAPUBIC ASPIRATION

INDICATIONS

Suprapubic aspiration (SPA) is one technique for obtaining an uncontaminated urine specimen in an infant (for alternatives, see below).

CONTRAINDICATIONS

It is futile to attempt the procedure if baby has just passed urine (i.e. the bladder is empty).

The bladder becomes a pelvic organ after the first year so SPA is not suitable after infancy.

EQUIPMENT

1. A 21 G or 23 G needle
2. A 5 ml syringe
3. Skin cleaning agent (alcohol wipe or fluid and gauze)
4. Cotton-wool ball
5. Adhesive plaster
6. Sterile container
7. Sterile gloves
8. Local anaesthetic cream (e.g. Emla)

PRE-PROCEDURAL CHECKS

Check all equipment. If the procedure is not urgent, apply local anaesthetic cream (under an occlusive dressing) to the lower abdomen about an hour beforehand. Check that the child can be held still in a supine position. Keep a sterile bowl to hand as abdominal palpation or skin preparation may induce urination and a 'clean catch' specimen can then be obtained.

TECHNIQUE

Cleanse the skin of the lower abdomen (between anterior superior iliac spines and the symphysis pubis). Attach the needle to the syringe.

Insert the needle perpendicularly to the skin 1 cm above the symphysis pubis to a depth of 1–3 cm, depending on the size of child. Aspirate as the needle is advanced and directed slightly caudally. If urine appears, continue aspirating. Then withdraw the needle. If no urine is aspirated, withdraw.

Occlude the entry site with a cotton-wool ball, and cover it with a plaster.

AFTERCARE

Cuddle the baby!

COMPLICATIONS

Fortunately, the technique is almost free from complications.

- A dry tap means that there is insufficient urine in the bladder. The attempt can be repeated after 2–3 h provided the baby does not pass urine in the meantime (ask the carer to watch and catch a 'clean catch' specimen if the infant urinates).
- Rarely, liquid faeces are aspirated from the colon. A single needle puncture of the bowel rarely causes any complication.
- Occasionally, a few red cells appear in the urine.

V

ALTERNATIVES

1. A 'clean catch' specimen would be appropriate for febrile children who are not seriously unwell but in whom a urinary tract infection must be excluded.
2. A specimen can be obtained by brief catheterization using a sterile procedure similar to that employed on adults. A small Foley catheter or nasogastric feeding tube can be used.

8. NASOGASTRIC TUBE INSERTION

INDICATIONS

Nasogastric tube insertion is indicated for:
  decompression of the stomach to reduce resistance to ventilation and
     the risk of regurgitation and aspiration
  giving drugs (e.g. activated charcoal)
  reduction of pain from gastric distension and easier assessment of the
     abdomen (e.g. in trauma)
  nasogastric feeding

CONTRAINDICATIONS

If a basal skull fracture is present (or is suspected clinically), then an orogastric tube must be considered instead.

EQUIPMENT

1. Appropriately sized nasogastric tube
2. Gloves
3. Lubricant gel and water
4. Tape to secure the tube
5. A 10 ml or 20 ml syringe
6. Litmus paper
7. Stethoscope
8. Drainage bag
9. Suction device

PRE-PROCEDURAL CHECKS

At least one assistant is required if the child is conscious. It may be easier for the assistant to cuddle and immobilize the child if small. Explain
the procedure to the carer beforehand and in an age-appropriate way

to the child. If unconscious and with an unprotected airway, the child should be on one side while the tube is being passed in case of vomiting. If the child is unconscious but airway reflexes are intact, the supine position with the neck in the position of 'sniffing the morning air' is helpful. In cases of trauma remember cervical spine immobilization technique. Check that all the equipment is ready.

TECHNIQUE

Measure and mark the tube for appropriate length by running it from the tip of the nose via the tragus of the ear to a midpoint between the xiphoid process and the umbilicus.

Lubricate the end of the tube with water or gel.

Pass the tube through the left or right nostril to the point marked on the tube. If the child is conscious, encourage repeated swallowing as you insert the tube.

Aim to pass the tube along the floor of the nostril and direct it straight back towards the occiput until it reaches the posterior pharyngeal wall; then attempt to direct it downwards.

Attach a syringe to the nasogastric tube and aspirate stomach contents. Beware that respiratory secretions may be aspirated. Check the pH of the secretions using litmus paper.

If no contents are aspirated, try injecting air into the tube and listen over the stomach with a stethoscope for a gurgling sound to confirm that the tube is in the stomach.

If the child vomits, becomes cyanosed, starts wheezing or choking, or experiences prolonged coughing fits, then the tube should be removed immediately as it has probably passed into the respiratory tract. Most commonly a misplaced tube will coil in the oropharynx.

Secure the tube with a piece of tape attached to the child's cheek.

Either aspirate the tube at regular intervals or leave it to drain freely.

AFTERCARE

Check that the tube is tolerated and mark it just below the nostril so that one can tell if it has become displaced. Always check that the tube is in the correct position before putting any fluid down it.

COMPLICATIONS

The nasogastric tube may pass into the left or right main bronchus as discussed above.

If a nasogastric tube is passed in a child with a basal skull fracture it may pass into the cranial cavity.

9. SPACER DEVICES AND INHALER TECHNIQUES

INDICATIONS

Even with optimal technique, deposition in the lungs of aerosol compounds from metered dose inhalers (MDIs) is inferior to that achieved with a spacer device. Whenever an MDI is prescribed, any child should always be encouraged to use it with a spacer device.

CONTRAINDICATIONS

There are no specific contraindications.

EQUIPMENT

1. Inhaler
2. Paediatric spacer, with mask

For children up to the age of 18 months, small spacer devices are available (Aerochamber, Babyhaler). Larger volume spacers (Volumatic, Nebuhaler) are appropriate for children of all ages but are more cumbersome. For children under 3 years old, the larger spacer devices may be prescribed as a 'Paediatric Volumatic' or 'Paediatric Nebuhaler' to ensure that they come with a face-mask.

It is important to know that the Volumatic is compatible with beclomethasone (Becotide) and salbutamol (Ventolin), as well as cromoglycate, fluticasone and salmeterol inhalers. The Nebuhaler is compatible with budesonide (Pulmicort) and terbutaline (Bricanyl). It makes no sense to prescribe different spacer systems for one child.

If a Volumatic spacer is used and the child is under 3 years old, the inspiratory effort may not be adequate to open the valve at the proximal end of the spacer. It is therefore common practice to push the valve out forcibly with a hard object such as a pen, although not included in Manufacturer's recommendations. If the valve has not been removed,

V

the distal end of the spacer can be angled above the proximal end (the mask) so that the valve is held open by gravity, allowing expiration alone to move it.

PRE-PROCEDURAL CHECKS

The spacer should be clean. The inhaler should not have exceeded its expiry date. The child should sit upright whenever possible, usually on the carer's lap.

TECHNIQUE

In children under 3 years old, the spacer should normally be used with a face-mask. Sometimes, children from the age of 2 years can accommodate the mouthpiece of the larger spacers and use them without the mask. Help the child and parents to experiment and find the best method.

When the mask is used, it should be attached to the spacer and applied firmly to the face (the Volumatic mask is very soft and pliable). The aerosol is discharged once into the spacer and 5–10 breaths or approximately 10 s of breathing is allowed. If more puffs are to be delivered, the procedure is repeated. The better the timing between puff and the inspiration the better the delivery of drug.

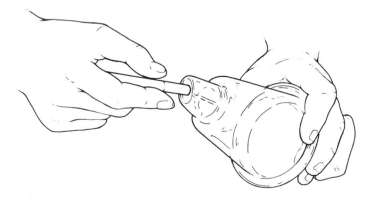

Fig. 28.9.1 *Removal of the valve from a spacer device. (Note warning in text.)*

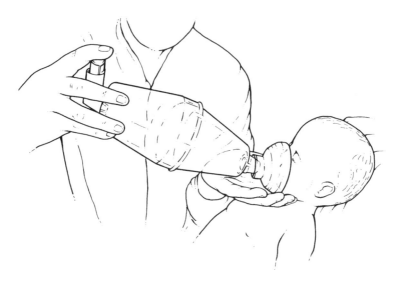

Fig. 28.9.2

The one puff and 5–10 breaths (or 10 s) technique can be repeated up to 10 times in the treatment of moderately severe asthma in the home or in hospital (total dose 10 × 100 µg = 1 mg salbutamol). This dose can be doubled, but failure to respond is then an indication for an urgent paediatric assessment.

> Careful explanation and demonstration of these techniques is of proven benefit in reducing the morbidity and number of hospital admissions for asthma.

V

AFTERCARE

The inhaler should be removed from the spacer and the mouth cover replaced to prevent dust entering.

The spacer and face-mask should be cleaned twice a week in a warm water. A mild detergent can be used. It is important to rinse the spacer thoroughly and allow to drip dry to avoid static electricity. If a film builds up inside, it can be removed with a soft toothbrush. The spacer should be replaced every 6 months.

COMPLICATIONS

Inadequate guidance and practice will result in inefficient use and a detrimental effect on asthma control.

10. REMOVAL OF FOREIGN BODY FROM EAR OR NOSE

INDICATIONS

Suspicion or history of foreign body insertion into the nose or ear canal.

CONTRAINDICATIONS

Any case for which there is a low probability of successful removal in the A&E department should be referred directly to the duty ENT speicalist, e.g. when the foreign body has been present for some time and visualization is impaired by chronic discharge.

EQUIPMENT

Some or all of the following equipment may be required and should be readily available.

1. Sedative medications if needed e.g. trimeprazine (see Chapter 25).
2. Means of immobilization: a sheet or (preferably) several assistants for holding the child
3. Auroscope
4. Nasal specula
5. Headlight (if experienced operator) or other light source
6. Topical vasoconstrictors, e.g. cocaine 4%, phenylephedrine 0.125%
7. Crocodile forceps
8. Wire loops, curettes
9. Suction apparatus, including catheters of various sizes
10. Blunt probes
11. A 30 ml or 60 ml syringe and suitable tubing

PRE-PROCEDURAL CHECKS

Ensure all equipment is readily to hand and that adequate lighting is available in the area to be used. Allow time for sedation to work if necessary. Ensure that the procedure is fully explained to the family and child (if appropriate). Ensure that immobilization is adequate before attempting removal. In the small child who cannot co-operate, at least one person should be assigned to hold the child's head and another to hold the limbs, with the child seated on the lap (or between the knees) of the carer or nurse.

TECHNIQUE

The myriad of methods advocated for the removal of aural and nasal foreign bodies bears testimony to the fact that none is universally successful. Local departmental guidelines should be followed where applicable. The following techniques have been successfully employed.

- Most nasal or aural foreign bodies can be removed by direct visualization and instrumentation through an auroscope.
- In experienced hands the use of nasal specula and a headlight are preferred for nasal foreign bodies; vertical opening of the specula will minimize septal damage.
- Topical vasoconstricor agents may reduce intranasal oedema and aid foreign body removal.
- Nasal foreign bodies usually lie on the nasal floor, lodged between the inferior turbinate and septum. A blunt instrument can be inserted over the object, which is then extracted against the nasal floor.
- Aural foreign bodies are best removed by the non-specialist by syringing; this includes insects, which are drowned. There is usually a gap between the posterosuperior canal and the object, so water should be aimed at the posterior canal wall to bypass the object and force it out after rebounding off the tympanic membrane. The water used should be at body temperature. A 30 ml or 60 ml syringe attached to a plastic infusion catheter or butterfly tubing (with the needle cut off) will produce adequate volumes of water at an appropriate pressure.

- Occasionally it is easier to remove aural foreign bodies with suction apparatus or a small Foley catheter, and this is a suitable alternative method. To avoid damage to the ear canal or tympanic membrane while using an auroscope the part of the hand holding the instrument should be rested against the child's head. If the child then moves suddenly, the examining hand and instrument will then move with the child's head.

AFTERCARE

After removal of the foreign body, remember to check the contralateral orifice. Check for trauma to mucosal surfaces. If there is significant trauma to the external ear canal consider prophylactic antibiotic therapy for acute otitis externa which is a common complication.

COMPLICATIONS

- The foreign body may be pushed into the nasopharynx from the nose and subsequently swallowed or aspirated.
- Local trauma – mucosal bleeding or oedema of the nose – is common.
- Tympanic membrane perforation can occur.
- Infection, typically otitis externa, can follow attempts at removal.
- Excessively forceful restraint can lead to ecchymoses in the child.

V

Failure of removal

Repeated attempts are unproductive. The following is recommended unless local guidelines exist:

- Nasal foreign body – refer to the duty ENT specialist.
- Aural foreign body – start the child on oral antibiotics (e.g. co-amoxiclav) and refer to the next ENT clinic.

11. FEMORAL NERVE BLOCK

INDICATIONS

Femoral nerve block is indicated to provide analgesia for femoral fracture. It can also be used for analgesia for injuries to the lower limb
(femoral nerve area) when assessment of other injuries would be
impeded by the use of systemic analgesia.

CONTRAINDICATIONS

No specific contraindication exists other than the practical difficulties
associated with the procedure (identification of correct site) or known
anaphylaxis to local anaesthetic agents.

EQUIPMENT

1. Local anaesthetic agents:
   bupivacaine 0.5% (1 ml per year of age up to 5 years old, 5 ml total
   for ages 5–12 years, 10 ml over 12 years)
   lignocaine 1%
2. Syringes (2 ml, 5 ml, 10 ml)
3. Needles (21 G and 25 G)
4. Gauze swabs
5. An assistant

PRE-PROCEDURAL CHECKS

It is vital to ensure everything is to hand and the affected limb is
positioned appropriately (with the affected limb gently abducted to
expose the groin).

TECHNIQUE

Identify the femoral artery and keep a finger applied to it.

The femoral nerve lies just lateral to the artery; the skin overlying can be anaesthetized using the 25 G needle and 2 ml syringe with lignocaine (if necessary).

Bupivacaine should then be injected around the nerve (after carefully aspirating to ensure the needle is not in the artery), using the 5 ml or 10 ml syringe and the 21 G needle.

AFTERCARE

Apply gentle pressure to the area to prevent bleeding and check adequacy of anaesthesia before further movement of the affected limb, after allowing a period of 20 min.

COMPLICATIONS

Complications may occur due to inadvertent injection of anaesthetic agent into artery or vein, which can be avoided using the technique above.

V

29 FRACTURES AND DISLOCATIONS

GENERAL PRINCIPLES

Fractures in children under 2 years old are uncommon, and non-accidental injury or bony pathology should be considered.

Any injury to the growth plate can potentially affect bone development producing deformity or shortening.

Dislocations and ligament injuries are more common in older children.

Children's bones are more flexible and this is responsible for buckle (torus) fractures and greenstick fractures (in which the cortex breaks on the side under tension but not on the compression side).

Remodelling is efficient in children and can be complete. It occurs most effectively in the plane of movement and is least effective at right angles to that plane, and with rotational injuries.

Children's fractures heal rapidly and any intervention should not therefore be unnecessarily delayed. In long-bone fractures, hyperaemia around the fracture site can increase bone growth during healing.

Neurovascular function must always be assessed distal to any fracture or dislocation.

Examination should follow the 'look, feel, and move' approach and be documented accordingly.

Undress the relevant limb and the opposite one for comparison.

Ensure that X-rays have been taken in at least two planes.

Do not forget to prescribe analgesics for all of the following injuries (see Chapter 25). Elevation also helps to relieve swelling and pain.

UPPER LIMB

CLAVICLE

Fractures of the clavicle commonly present with loss of upper limb function. The clavicle must always be inspected and palpated in these children. Clavicular fractures are rarely open and neurovascular injuries or pneumothorax are rare. Support in a sling is the standard treatment (or collar and cuff if the sling is uncomfortable).

SCAPULA

Fractures of the scapula are rare in children. Early intervention is necessary when the glenoid is involved. Scapular fractures are associated with underlying rib and visceral chest injuries.

HUMERUS

Exclude radial nerve or other neurovascular trauma. Refer any displaced injury directly to orthopaedic staff. Minimally displaced fractures of the humeral neck or shaft can be treated with dependent traction in a collar and cuff, supplemented by a body bandage for support.

SUPRACONDYLAR FRACTURE

Displaced supracondylar fractures pose a risk of brachial artery compression and they require orthopaedic assessment and manipulation. Undisplaced fractures can be treated in a high collar and cuff, with or without an above-elbow backslab, as long as there is no neurovascular compromise (check the wrist pulses and the capillary circulation).

OTHER FRACTURES AROUND THE ELBOW

Undisplaced fractures may be treated with a collar and cuff, but referral is necessary for displaced fractures which usually require surgery.

PULLED ELBOW

See Chapter 15.

ELBOW DISLOCATION

Dislocation of the elbow is rare in children. Check neurovascular function which may be impaired. Refer to orthopaedic staff on-call.

FOREARM FRACTURES

Check that these are not associated with dislocation of the radial or ulnar heads (the Monteggia and Galeazzi injuries respectively). A vertical line through the radial head must cross the capitulum of the distal radius. Displaced forearm fractures and associated dislocations must be referred for manipulation. Undisplaced fractures can be treated with an above-elbow backslab and referred to the fracture clinic.

FRACTURES OF THE DISTAL RADIUS

Minor buckle fractures are common and require nothing more than protection in a plaster for approximately 2 weeks. Angulated greenstick or other displaced fractures will require manipulation under general anaesthesia, although regional or local anaesthesia may be tolerated in patients over the age of about 12 years.

CARPAL FRACTURES

Carpal fractures are rare in children. The scaphoid fractures which are occasionally seen in older children should be immobilized in a standard scaphoid cast.

HAND FRACTURES

Angulated, rotated and other displaced fractures involving joint surfaces require direct orthopaedic referral. Undisplaced buckle or epiphyseal fractures (usually of the proximal phalanx) require nothing more than strapping of adjacent fingers.

CRUSH INJURIES OF THE FINGERTIPS

Fractures of the tuft of the distal phalanx are technically open (if there is a breach of the skin) and broad-spectrum antistaphylococcal antibiotics are recommended. These injuries are common (they usually result from being trapped in a door) but they heal very well in children; such injuries should be dressed regularly (e.g. twice weekly) and observed for spontaneous healing.

LOWER LIMB

PELVIC FRACTURES

Unstable fractures of the pelvic ring result from serious trauma, and accompanying visceral injuries and hypovolaemic shock (usually from retroperitoneal bleeding) are associated with a high mortality rate. Surgical and orthopaedic referrals are indicated.

An injury specific to children is epiphyseal avulsion (e.g. of the iliac crest or spine) which usually requires nothing more than conservative treatment. All pelvic fractures should be referred.

FRACTURES AROUND THE HIP

Fractures around the hip are uncommon in children but dislocations and fractures of the femoral neck can produce avascular necrosis of the femoral head. All require direct referral.

V

FEMORAL FRACTURES

Femoral fractures must be referred but skin traction can be applied temporarily in the A&E department.

FRACTURES AROUND THE KNEE

Injuries to the epiphyseal plate of the distal femur may only be suspected by focal tenderness and X-rays can appear normal unless the
limb is stressed. All displaced fractures around the knee should be
referred. Undisplaced injuries can be treated with a split plaster cylinder
and weight can then be kept off and the limb elevated until the child
has been seen in the fracture clinic. A plaster check for neurovascular
function is important the following day. In children, avulsion of the
anterior cruciate attachment (tibial spine) is more common than rupture of the substance of the ligament. It is also more easily treated by
reattachment.

PATELLAR DISLOCATION

The diagnosis is often made retrospectively when the patella relocates
as the knee is extended. If not, the lateral situation of the patella is diagnostic and reduction is achieved by administering analgesia and gently
straightening the knee while applying pressure to the lateral side of the
patella. General anaesthesia is not normally required, and as the injury
is most common in teenagers, light sedation and nitrous oxide inhalation is more easily administered. Chip fractures of the patella may result
from the shearing force and an intra-articular loose body can result, so
X-rays must be obtained.

TIBIAL FRACTURES

Undisplaced tibial fractures may be treated in an above-knee, full-
length split backslab, elevated, and referred to the fracture clinic. A
plaster check the following day is important. Displaced injuries need to
be referred directly. Stress fractures should also be immobilized in
plaster.

ANKLE FRACTURES

Undisplaced malleolar fractures should be immobilized in a below-knee plaster and the patient referred to the fracture clinic. Displaced injuries require an orthopaedic opinion at the time.

FOOT FRACTURES

Foot fractures are uncommon, except with metatarsal injuries, which may be supported in a below-knee cast if strapping or bandaging gives inadequate support.

V

PART VI

Useful Data

FACTS AND FIGURES

WEIGHT

Weight in kg = 2 × (age in years + 4)

Note:

    infant weight gain 30 g per day from 10th day
    birthweight × 2 by age 5 months
    birthweight × 3 by age 1 year

ENERGY REQUIREMENTS

- Up to 1 year old: 460 kJ (110 kcal) per day for each kg of body weight, up to 590 kJ (140 kcal) per day for premature infants.
- Remember – 150 ml milk contains 460 kJ (110 kcal).

BLOOD VOLUME

- Child over 1 year old:
  blood volume in ml = 80 × weight in kg
- Under 1 year old:
  blood volume in ml = (80 to 100) × weight in kg

BASIC OBSERVATIONS

Age (years)	Respiratory rate (min^{-1})	Systolic BP (mmHg)	Pulse
<1	30–40	70–90	110–160
2–5	23–30	80–100	95–140
5–12	20–25	90–110	80–120
>12	15–20	100–120	60–100

VI

FLUID REQUIREMENTS

- Maintenance fluids – use dextrose saline (sodium chloride 0.18%, glucose 4%) unless otherwise indicated in guidance notes.

- See table below for fluid volumes.

Weight of child	Fluid per 24 h (ml kg^{-1})	Fluid per h (ml kg^{-1})	Na$^+$ per 24 h (mmol kg^{-1})	K$^+$ per 24 h (mmol kg^{-1})
First 10 kg	100	4	2–4	1.5–2.5
Second 10 kg	50	2	1–2	0.5–1.5
Thereafter	20	1	0.5–1	0.2–0.7

VENTILATION

	Expected Peak Flow Values	
Height (cm)	Very approximate age (years)	Peak flow (l min^{-1})
110	5–6	150
120	6–7	200
130	7–8	250
140	8–10	300
150	10–12	350
160	12–14	400
170	14+	450

Intubation

- Appropriate size of endotracheal tube:
  Internal diameter (mm) = (age/4) + 4
  Length (cm) = (age/2) + 12 for an oral tube
  Length (cm) = (age/2) + 15 for a nasal tube
  Where ages are in years.

ASSESSMENT OF CONSCIOUS LEVEL

- The children's coma scale should be used in children < 4 years old.
- The Glasgow coma scale should be used in older children.

Glasgow coma scale (4–15 years)		Children's coma scale (< 4 years)	
Response	Score	Response	Score
EYES		EYES	
Open spontaneously	4	Open spontaneously	4
Verbal command	3	React to speech	3
React to pain	2	React to pain	2
No response	1	No response	1
BEST MOTOR RESPONSE		BEST MOTOR RESPONSE	
Obeys verbal command	6	Spontaneous or obeys verbal command	6
Painful stimulus		*Painful stimulus*	
Localizes pain	5	Localizes pain	5
Flexion with pain	4	Withdraws in response to pain	4
Flexion abnormal	3	Abnormal flexion to pain	3
Extension	2	(decorticate posture)	
No response	1	Abnormal extension to pain	2
		(decerebrate posture)	
		No response	1
BEST VERBAL RESPONSE		BEST VERBAL RESPONSE	
Orientated and converses	5	Smiles, orientated to sounds, follows objects, interacts	5
Disorientated and converses	4	*Crying* (baby) *Interacts* (child)	
Inappropriate words	3	Consolable Inappropriate	4
Incomprehensible sounds	2	Inconsistently	
No response	1	consolable Moaning	3
		Inconsolable Irritable	2
		No response No response	1
The total of the score in each of the three sections is the coma scale score			

VI

INDEX

Note – Page numbers in **bold type** refer to tables and boxes